# DIASTASIS RECTI

## SECRETS

### FOR NEW MOMS

Proven Methods and
Postpartum Exercises
for healing core weakness
and weight loss

## BECKY CHOI

# DIASTASIS RECTI SECRETS FOR NEW MOMS

*Proven Methods and Postpartum Exercises for*
*Healing Core Weakness and Weight Loss*

*By*

# Becky Choi

Thank you for downloading the Diastasis Recti Secrets for New Moms e-book.

Sign up for our exclusive video exercise series and references mentioned in the book to heal your diastasis quicker.

Visit us online at guide.beckychoi.com

More bite-sized resources available here on Instagram

www.instagram.com/beckychoi

* * *

If you like this book, your review on Amazon kindle will inspire thousands of moms just like you who are stuck and feeling uncomfortable about themselves. I hope you can continue the Tummy Warrior movement and guide them to the light.

Review and rate this book now.

Diastasis Recti Secrets for New Moms

Proven Methods and Postpartum Exercises for Healing Core Weakness and Weight Loss

## Legal Notice and Disclaimer

## Qualifications

Becky Choi is a Certified Postpartum Corrective Exercise Specialist, and she holds a certificate in Personal Training, and that is the extent of her medical and professional certifications related to Diastasis Recti. Becky Choi makes no representations to hold any other qualifications or certifications outside of this. Becky Choi recommends you seek a medical professional should you have any questions about any content on this book and before taking any actions related to content you may read on this book.

## Not Professional Advice

Nothing shared in this book by Becky Choi is professional advice. This is simply a compilation of things Becky Choi has learned through her own experiences and studying to be a Certified

Postpartum Corrective Exercise Specialist and Personal Trainer. Nothing in this book is professional advice.

## No Guarantees

You understand that Becky Choi makes no guarantees whatsoever regarding any results based on any action or inaction relating to your health, fitness, body or Diastasis Recti based on the information we share or services we sell or share for free through this book. At the end of the day, we will not be responsible or make any promises for what will happen in your life and health.

## Releasing Becky Choi of Liability

Becky Choi will not be liable for any actions you do or not take based on the information on this book. Becky Choi will not be liable and responsible for any form of damages or any legal claims against it for any damages based on your participation and application in using this book.

# Table of Contents

# Acknowledgement

A special thank you to my family.

Thank you, my husband Dan, for being the most supportive husband I can ever dream of. None of this would happen without your unconditional loving support.

Thank you, my two adorable children, Jordan and Emily, for coming into my life. Your smiles, laughter and affection have lit my soul on fire. Every moment is packed with gratitude.

> *'Jordan and Emily, follow your dreams and dream BIG. Don't settle for anything less than your goals. You have the power, strength and all the resources available. Don't worry, Mommy will be a living example for you.'*

**– Mommy**

# Foreword

Every mother has her own unique version of the ancient saga called Motherhood. It consumes, overwhelms, transforms, fulfills and redefines us, our relationships, our whole lives. It turns out to be everything you imagined it would be, and somehow, also the exact opposite. Loving was never so easy, nor doing ever so hard. Those first few newborn months are especially emotional with relentless pushing and pulling. And in that tizzy, you get immense comfort when you hear another mom's story and feel, 'Yes! That's exactly how I feel too. I'm not alone in this after all.'

This is precisely how I felt while reading *this* book.

A few months ago, I discovered that I have severe diastasis recti. And I've probably had it since I had my first baby four years ago. No doctor, no friend, no pregnancy or baby book ever told me about this. I went on to have another baby last year, and probably decimated my abdominal wall. More than a year postpartum, I still had a five-month belly and hated my body. One fretful night, trawling through the rabbit hole of the internet, I chanced upon 'diastasis recti'. I checked my gap immediately, and voila! I'd found my answer!

I spent the next several weeks earnestly reading blogs, social media posts, watching videos, doing 21-day DR challenges, 10-day core bootcamps etc. etc. And nothing. My gap was the same and I didn't lose an inch off my tummy. I was so confused, so desperate and so alone.

I now know that I was far from alone. Nearly a third of all new mothers suffer from diastasis recti that doesn't heal itself. Ideally, your doctor or midwife should tell you all about it, but clearly, that's not happening yet. Lots of women just accept this as the 'mummy tummy' and struggle to restore their core. There is a huge knowledge gap that exists here, and lately, there has been a welcome increase in this conversation on the social media. But it's fairly challenging to separate the wheat from the chaff on social media. There is very little comprehensive, accessible and research-backed information out there.

Becky Choi's *Diastasis Recti Secrets for New Moms*, is a big step in the right direction.

Becky brings together her personal experience of diastasis recti with her deep interest in postpartum fitness to provide a unique solution to this surprisingly common condition. She understands the challenges of balancing your life as a mother, while wanting to take care of yourself, heal your diastasis recti, and get the hell out of your oversized, maternity clothes.

Through lots of trial, error and research, Becky finally found a way to lose her pregnancy weight, strengthen her core, tone her abs, *and* heal her severe diastasis recti. She has integrated all her learnings to build the Tummy Warrior Method to help fellow moms like you and me.

*Diastasis Recti Secrets for New Moms* takes the reader on a step-by-step journey of understanding and healing her diastasis recti. It delves into the Tummy Warrior Method, explaining its seven steps in generous detail. Full of examples, illustrations and useful little tips, it will help you make the right exercise and nutrition choices that, very importantly, fit into your existing lifestyle. It goes beyond the one-size-fits-all approach, and empowers you with the knowledge and tools to become your own coach. And not in the least, it brings into focus the game-changing impact of deep breathing, and the vast rewards of consistent practice.

Having been a Tummy Warrior myself, I know that this pursuit that you are on is not an easy one. *Diastasis Recti Secrets for New Moms* breaks down this daunting process, bringing a fit, strong, and healthy body within the reach of the readers who refuse to accept the status quo and seek to feel confident in their beautiful bodies again.

**Shradha Biyani**
**September 2020**

# Section One:

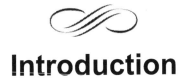

# Introduction

# Chapter 1:

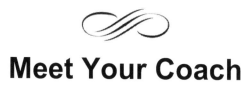

## Meet Your Coach

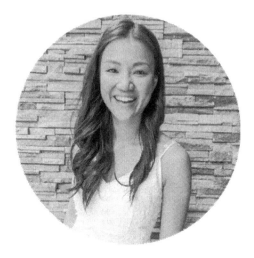

*Hi! My name is Becky Choi. I am so glad you are here!*

Four years ago, I was a new mom who had just had her first baby boy, my beautiful Jordan. As a first-time mom, I was filled with joy and excitement. He was perfect! I kissed his little feet all day long, snuggled with him skin to skin, and like most parents, took a lot of pictures of him! But I rarely took pictures of us together because I couldn't stand the way I looked in photos. I gained over 40 lbs during my pregnancy, and even after giving birth I remained heavier 25 lbs than my pre-pregnancy weight.

Every time I looked in the mirror, I wanted to punch it because I hated what I saw. I was the biggest I had ever been, and I had a huge belly. I wanted to get back into my pre-baby shape to fit into my old jeans and snug dresses. Even though I wished to lose weight, I had never worked out before so I didn't know where to begin. I constantly felt self-conscious, even in front of my husband and child. I felt like I was weighing the whole family down with my body image issues.

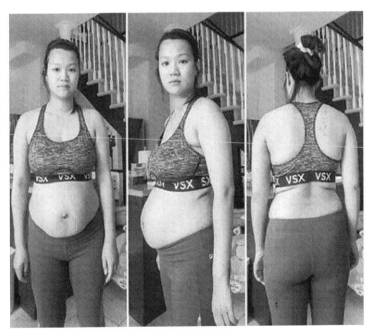

*September 2016 , 3 months postpartum*

Then my husband, who likes working out, introduced me to a high-intensity full-body workout program, which had cardio and strength training and yoga all rolled into one. It was challenging but fun, and I could do it at home.

After a few months of following that, I lost 20 lbs, but I still had an enormous belly that made me look five months pregnant all the time. I was so frustrated because I thought that if I lost the extra weight, I would lose the belly fat too.

Later, I was diagnosed with severe Diastasis Recti, which meant that my core muscles had been overly stretched, creating a vertical squishy space in the middle of my abs. It is a surprisingly common condition caused by childbearing. It turned out that my large belly wasn't just layers of fat after all. My family doctor recommended cosmetic surgery, but not if I still wanted to have more kids, and I did.

I remember looking at my pre-pregnancy dresses collecting dust in the closet. I took them out and laid them out on the bed, so I could take a final look and reminisce about the good times I had wearing them. Then I started stuffing everything into a box like a madwoman. I donated all of them because I felt so lost and hopeless. I thought that I was never going to fit into them again, and I just had to accept the fact that I'd always carry a huge belly.

Soon I was pregnant again, and a little under a year later, I gave birth to my baby girl. I had piled on the pounds again. At six weeks postpartum, I visited a local physiotherapist. She was knowledgeable about diastasis recti, and taught me how to engage my deep core muscles, how to implement DR-specific exercises and what things I should be mindful of.

The thing was, I was 25 lbs overweight. With two kids now, I wanted to feel lighter and have more energy to care for them. Most importantly, I didn't want to chase after two kids and aggravate my health conditions due to the severe diastasis. All of a sudden, I had a light bulb moment! What if I combined the DR exercises with the same high-intensity full-body workouts I did after my first baby? If I didn't know that I had diastasis recti and still managed to lose 20 lbs, then it could not be any worse this time.

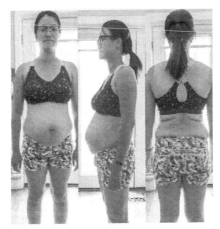

*August 2018, 15 weeks postpartum*

I started swapping anything I could not handle in the high-intensity workouts with my DR exercises, but still followed most of the training. I slowly figured out that gassy foods can cause bloating, so I implemented a new nutrition regime. I also wore a belly wrap which helped with my posture, and was a massive support for my workout and daily activities.

I lost a lot of weight, and my core seemed to be getting stronger. In fact, my diastasis measurement was down from 4.5 fingers wide to 1 finger wide. But appearance-wise, the belly was still very visible. I remember standing up and looking down to my toes, but I couldn't see them because my belly was blocking the view. I was disappointed that my tummy was still so big, but I knew that I was moving in the right direction. I told myself if I had already come this far, I am not giving up. Seven months later, I consulted another women's health physiotherapist, Munira Hudani.

Then, I studied intensively on the topics of Diastasis Recti, including a course instructed by Dr. Sarah Duvall. With their guidance, my experience, and the new knowledge, I took a few steps back.

I went back to the basics and focused my attention on breathing, engaging the deep core muscle, and aligning my body while doing the high-intensity full-body workout. I looked back at the mistakes I made and started to make sense of what I could improve on. I started slowly, but those seemingly small changes ushered in the significant results.

I lost 35 lbs, and have maintained it since. I trimmed 10 inches off my waist. I am the strongest and lightest that I have ever been. My core is healing well. And it feels incredible to be able to fit into a dress and not look pregnant finally!

Fitness has become an essential part of my lifestyle now. In fact, I recently resigned from my job at the bank where I worked for over ten years, to pursue my passion in postpartum fitness, and formally trained to become a diastasis recti specialist. It feels incredible to bring my experience and knowledge to empower moms like you who are reading this book. And I am so proud to have created a community of like-minded women, The Tummy Warriors. It is humbling to be able to motivate, lead and inspire them, so they feel confident and beautiful in their bodies.

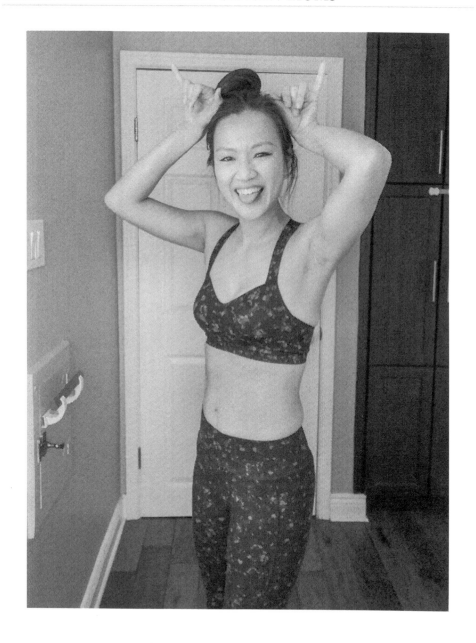

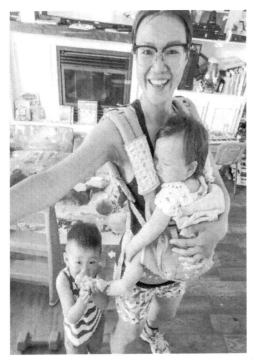

*My cheerleaders while I worked out in the living room, they are the reason that kept me going. Thank you Jordan and Emily.*

# Chapter 2:

# Preparation Work

### Diastasis Recti Secrets

I am excited to share my secrets with you in these pages! My guess is that this is probably not your first time reading about diastasis recti. And if you've failed at trying to get rid of the mummy tummy despite your efforts, please know that it is not your fault. There is a lot of information out there, and it can be confusing. Very often, excessive and unstructured information keeps you from getting the desired results. But it's not the end of the road. I want to reassure you that you are in the right place.

If you've reached the point where you feel like you have tried everything, but you just didn't see any difference, I want you to put those fears and worries to rest. I do not doubt that you will reach your goals when you follow the seven secrets I reveal in this book. I have seen many success stories in our community, and you can be one of them. You can do this!

The majority of the resources online and some trainers will probably tell you to do gentle, diastasis recti-safe exercises and avoid many things. Some will ask you to do only a few types of core rehab workcuts, and some, unfortunately, have no idea what they are talking about. There are so many approaches to this, and everyone has their own opinions. Some of it might even work to some extent, but healing severe diastasis recti needs a deeper understanding of the condition and our bodies.

I truly do care about your success because I have been exactly where you are. I know how it feels when you stand in front of your closet in despair, feeling like you have nothing to wear. When you have to cut the elastic band of your shorts, so you can fit in it. When you're no longer pregnant but still have to wear your maternity clothes. And the worst is, when people ask you, 'When are you due?' So many times, I've wanted to dig a hole and hide. I understand entirely how that destroys your self-esteem, and affects your relationship with your partner.

Many of the trainers you come across have no personal experience of this journey. Some have never given birth, or some did but did not have severe diastasis recti. Some of them fixed their bellies with tummy tuck surgeries. They teach you based on theory, based on what other people have been doing in the last decade, and that knowledge gap is why their exercises aren't entirely effective. They don't understand what it is really like when you are in the trenches.

The feeling of dejection when you measure the same after weeks of working out or dieting. The utterly lonesome feeling. The feeling that why only me? Why none of my friends? Why does nobody know what is going on?!

Mama, I am here to tell you, you are not alone. I am with you. You deserve to feel beautiful and confident in your own skin. And I know you can rock your jeans and bathing suits. You just need to get on the right path.

Are you ready for the secrets?

## What is Diastasis Recti (DR)?

The term 'diastasis recti' or 'diastasis recti abdominis' sounds so esoteric. Like a secret code you need to use the loo in a spacecraft. Most moms had not heard of diastasis recti until recent years. However, every mom should be aware of what DR is, because it is so common.

In fact, a study has found that 100 per cent of women who carry till full-term experience DR around their due date. In more than half the women the DR heals itself, but a research study found that at 6 months postpartum 39 per cent of women still have DR, and at 12 months postpartum it's still 32 per cent.

So, about one-third of all moms live with diastasis recti for who knows how long!

Diastasis recti is caused when the stomach muscles have been overly stretched and weakened to make room for the growing baby during pregnancy. Although diastasis recti is most common in postpartum women, it can also happen in men or women from working out too hard or using improper techniques or gaining weight drastically.

During pregnancy, as the baby grows, the linea alba (Figure 2.1) stretches like an elastic band, along with the entire abdominal wall to make room. The expansion is due to an excessive rise in intra-abdominal pressure and hormonal changes.

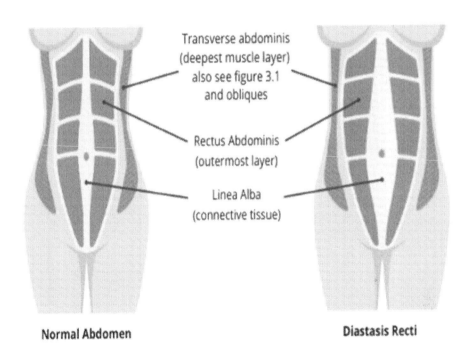

Transverse abdominis
(deepest muscle layer)
also see figure 3.1
and obliques

Rectus Abdominis
(outermost layer)

Linea Alba
(connective tissue)

Normal Abdomen                    Diastasis Recti

*Figure 2.1*

Sometimes the abdominal wall gets too stretched and thinned out, and doesn't go back to its initial state after the baby is delivered. In doing so, it often causes other organs such as the intestines to be pushed around and hang forward making your belly protrude more. If it is not healed correctly, it can cause problems after birth, both physically and emotionally. Many women often call this a 'pooch'. And some describe their appearance as if they are still several months pregnant.

Additionally, because the abdominal muscles are compromised, a woman can experience constipation, incontinence, and lower back pain. These occur because the muscles in this region are weakened, causing more reliance on other tissues, and can be aggravated by poor posture and improper breathing.

Worst yet, you could develop a hernia or experience a pelvic organ prolapse. A hernia happens when an organ pushes through an opening in the muscle or the tissue that holds it in place. For example, an umbilical hernia is when the intestine protrudes through the umbilical opening in the abdominal muscles. With hernia, you will usually see a round bulge near the navel. We will discuss hernia and pelvic floor dysfunction in section 3.

## How to Measure Diastasis Recti

If you have given birth recently, please allow yourself to rest and don't worry about it for now. For the first six weeks, your body and especially your tummy is in a healing phase. You may unintentionally worsen it if you do crunch-like diastasis recti check. C-section mommies may need a few extra weeks.

When your doctor clears you for exercise, it is recommended that you see a women's health physiotherapist for a thorough check-up. If you can't, then here is how you can do a self-check to measure your diastasis. There are three areas point 1, 2, and 3 on figure 2.2 that you will be checking on yourself.

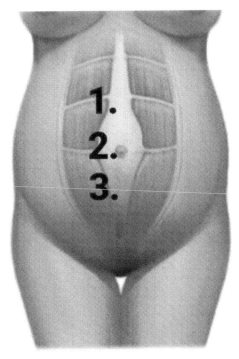

*Figure 2.2*

1. Check first thing in the morning, before you eat or drink anything, because your tummy is at its flattest, and the

connective tissue hasn't expanded yet with your daily activities.

2. Lie on your back with your knees bent and feet flat on the floor.

3. Inhale and exhale as you lift your head up just slightly off the floor, moving your chin towards your chest.

Begin by putting your fingers in the middle and gently press down on Point 1. How many fingers can you fit between the muscles? How deep can you sink your finger in i.e. how many knuckles? Write that down.

Repeat for points 2 and 3.

The finger gap between your external core muscles determines how severe your diastasis is. How far your finger can sink in determines how weak your connective tissue linea alba is (Figure 2.1). For example, I could fit almost five fingers between my muscles in the beginning, and I could sink two knuckles into the tissue.

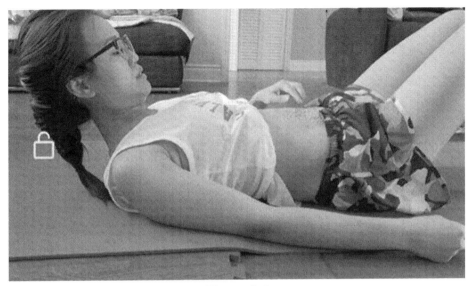

*Figure 2.3*

It's important to note that you can have a three-fingers gap but still have a strong core. A strong core means that your linea alba can maintain tension or contain the intra-abdominal pressure even when you move around and exercise. In other words, your core is functional. Your belly may or may not appear flat. Vice versa, you could have a two fingers wide gap but a weak core, so the internal organs can easily hang forward when you are upright because the core muscles are not strong enough to hold them in place. In this case, you will have a pregnant looking belly. You may also see doming (we will talk about doming in a moment).

| Finger | Severity |
|--------|----------|
| 1 finger | Normal |
| 2-3 fingers | Mild |
| 3-4 fingers | Mild/ Severe |
| 4+ fingers | Severe |

*Figure 2.4*

For quick reference, this chart determines the severity of your diastasis recti initially. However, rest assured that you can have a strong core with a three-fingers wide gap.

## How to Treat Diastasis Recti

This is the reason why I wrote this book! And here is where I reveal my secrets. We can heal our DR and strengthen our core by following these seven steps in sequence. Our goal is not just to close the gap, but also to restore the normal functioning of the abdominal wall, so we can get a strong core. And in doing so, we get a flat stomach, a happy by-product of a strong core. I am also going to show you how you can lose weight while healing the diastasis recti at the same time so that you can get into the best shape of your life. Yes, even better than before you had your baby!

This book is your secret manual no matter where you are at in your journey. And the seven secrets are:

1. Transverse Abdominis Engagement,

2. Posture Matters,

3. A Belly Wraps,

4. Tension,

5. High-Intensity Total Body Workouts,

6. Diastasis Recti Nutrition, and

7. Consistency

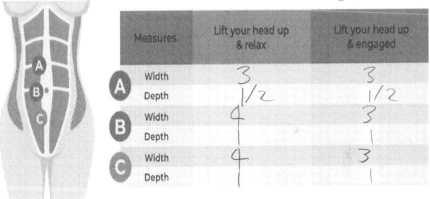

**DR MEASUREMENT**
**BEFORE**

| | Measures | Lift your head up & relax | Lift your head up & engaged |
|---|---|---|---|
| A | Width | 3 | 3 |
| A | Depth | 1/2 | 1/2 |
| B | Width | 4 | 3 |
| B | Depth | 1 | 1 |
| C | Width | 4 | 3 |
| C | Depth | 1 | 1 |

*Figure 2.5: Take Your Diastasis Recti Measurement Now*

## DR MEASUREMENT
## AFTER

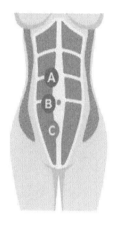

| Measures | | Lift your head up & relax | Lift your head up & engaged |
|---|---|---|---|
| **A** | Width | | |
| | Depth | | |
| **B** | Width | | |
| | Depth | | |
| **C** | Width | | |
| | Depth | | |

# Section Two:

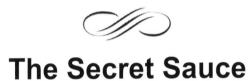

# The Secret Sauce

# Chapter 3:

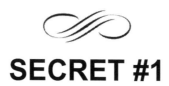

# SECRET #1

## Transverse Abdominis Engagement

Before you learn how to engage your TA, it is essential to take a moment to understand the different parts of your core. Most people may think of abs as the six-pack muscles, and though that is a part of your core, there is much more to your core than that. A whole set of muscles and tissues together form your core, and you rely on them heavily for your day-to-day activities – whether you are picking up your child or lifting a bag full of groceries, reaching for a dish on a high shelf, or even getting in and out of bed. Even when you cough and sneeze or laugh really hard, you are using your core!

## The Foundation: The Transverse Abdominal Muscle

The transverse abdominal muscle (TA) is like a corset of deepest inner core muscles that wrap around from the front of your abdomen all the way to the back. At the top, it interconnects with the diaphragm. And at the bottom, it inserts into the pubic symphysis.

As I've mentioned earlier, the key difference between my first and second postpartum experience was that I did not know initially that I had diastasis recti. Therefore, I didn't learn how to breathe and engage the TA muscles properly. That's why, even though I exercised consistently and lost 20 lbs, the gap and doming were still extremely prominent. Due to the improper exercise techniques, I had worsened my diastasis condition unintentionally.

Knowing how to breathe and activate your TA is crucial to the healing process. Without this step, all the other steps are pointless. And frankly, a lot of people do not know that they have diastasis recti, and then they join mommy's boot camp and start working out without the proper techniques.

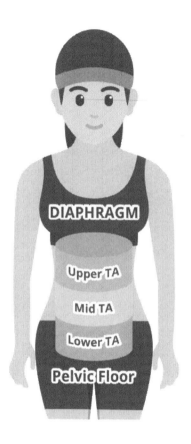

*Figure 3.1: The Core Canister Anatomy*

In this image, figure 3.1, it is the anatomy of your core which I refer to as a core canister. I would like to quickly give you an overview of where your diaphragm, transverse abdominal muscles and pelvic floor are visually.

The top of the canister is your diaphragm.

The bottom of the canister is your pelvic floor.

The back of the canister is your back muscle or the multifidus.

The inner part of the canister is your transverse abdominal muscle which is a corset muscle that wraps around your core, there is an upper TA, mid-TA and lower TA

The front of the canister is the rectus abdominal muscle which is the six-pack.

You also have obliques (internal and external; on the side).

Take a moment and give some thoughts to where your muscles are located. We are going to refer back to this canister from time to time throughout this book.

## Deep Breathing

When you inhale deeply, your lungs fill with air, your diaphragm expands downward, your pelvic floor is relaxed, your ribs expand, and your back muscles, chest and belly expand. The breath distributes evenly into your system like opening up an upside-down umbrella. Or at least, this is what should happen when you breathe mindfully and deeply.

When you exhale, the diaphragm and pelvic floor rise up, and the air is pushed out of the lungs.

However, one of the biggest issues that happen during pregnancy, and often continues postpartum, is that your breath either becomes shallow i.e. goes only into your chest and shoulders, or you become a belly breather in which too much air goes into your belly making it rise and fall excessively. Some of your muscles become imbalanced and are unable to function normally. In order to engage our transverse abdominal muscle once again, you must relearn how to breathe properly by connecting your mind to your inner body.

## Transverse Abdominal Muscles Engagement with 360 Breathing

I would like to invite you to work alongside me in the following pages. You will practice engaging your TA in these four positions:

1. Lying on your back.
2. Sitting on a chair.
3. Standing.
4. Lying on your side.

## Practice Together

Lie down on your back, either on the floor or on your bed. We will work on three areas (figure 3.2).

Before we start, take a deep breath and send your breath to the sides of your ribs, the back and the belly as you take a deep inhale. As you inhale, your pelvic floor should be relaxed without any pressure.

You should watch yourself in a mirror if you can, or use your phone to record yourself as you inhale. First, your full-back should be touching the floor with no arch. Second, when you inhale, ask yourself "does the inhale go straight down to my belly, blowing it up like a balloon? Or does the breath only go to my upper chest area?" The breath needs to be distributed equally, you should feel that your sides, back and belly expand equally at the same time. This is what I call '360-degree breathing' or just '360 breathing' for short.

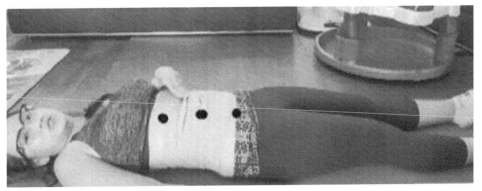

*Figure 3.2*

## Start with the Belly Button

Put your hands on either side on your belly. Inhale 360 degrees. Imagine the three and nine on a clock are trying to meet in the middle where your belly button is. As you exhale, make a 'shhh...'

sound and gently pull your belly button down towards the spine. One thing I want you to watch out for here is that, when you pull your belly button down towards the spine, your lower belly does not pop up filling with pressure. If it does, then lessen the degree of pulling your belly button inward so your stomach is evenly flat.

## Below the Belly Button

Here we will work on a few inches below the navel where the pelvic bones are. If you are familiar with doing Kegels (you will learn about Kegels in Section 3 of the book), it is a similar approach. Our pelvic floor and abdominal muscles work closely together. You can also imagine that you are trying to stop the flow of urine or picking up a marble with your lady parts. Relax the belly, take a slow deep inhale, and exhale slowly as you imagine your lady parts picking the marble up towards your belly button. To stay focused on your exhale, you can exhale through your mouth or say 'shhhh...' or make a 'haaa...' sound. Exhale slowly until all the air is out, and don't let go of your pelvic floor muscles until you start your next inhale.

## Above the Belly Button

Repeat this inhale-exhale one more time a few inches above the navel. But this time imagine your left and right rib cages are drawing together in the middle. You should use your hands to guide you. Take a deep 360 inhale, and then exhale with an audible 'haaa...'

sound, and 'haaa...' very slowly until nothing is left in your lungs. It should be about five to ten seconds of 'ha-ing'.

Once you are comfortable with activating the TA lying on your back, try doing the inhale-exhale while sitting and standing in front of a mirror. When you are in the sitting or standing position, focus on activating the area below the navel where the pelvic bones are. The breathing exercises are the same as above.

A quick tip that I learnt from Munira Hudani, women's health physiotherapist, to see whether you are rightly activating your lower TA, is to draw in the belly in slow motion, and pay attention to the belly button. Check to see whether your belly button is sliding upwards. Can you see your upper abs suck inward before your lower abs? You don't want that to happen as your goal is to isolate other muscles and only use your lower TA. Think of activating your TA with a bottom-up approach. First, your pelvic floor fires up, then your lower abs, then your mid abs and finally your upper abs. Your belly button should go straight in instead of sliding upwards. This is what you want to achieve when you engage your belly button and below your belly button TA.

If you do not see this bottom-up pattern, it probably means that you aren't activating the right muscles. You are still doing the work, but it won't be as effective. In this case, you may have to try another position such as standing or lying on your sides. The goal here is to be comfortable activating your deep core muscles on demand throughout the day, especially when you exercise or exert yourself.

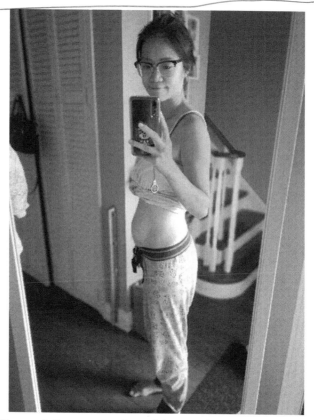

*Figure 3.3: practice breathing in front of the mirror*

You will need to get comfortable in activating your TA in all four positions. A lot of the work is subtle and internal. It is not hard physical labour like a high-intensity workout, and you may not feel like it is doing anything. Therefore, I find that this is the most commonly ignored exercise.

Please do not skip this step. It is normal to not feel too much, especially in the beginning when you have never done the breathing exercises. This is a mind-to-muscle connection, and calls for more mental awareness than physical work.

You may have gotten disconnected from how you used to breathe before pregnancy. But as long as you are following the cues on the next few pages, you are going to get better at it. Whether you've only just discovered you have DR, or you have been exercising for a while, you need to make sure you know how to engage your TA in all four positions.

## Common Mistakes When Activating the Transverse Abdominis

When you practice the TA activation while standing up or sitting on a chair, you should do it in front of a mirror and pay attention to your ribs. Do you see your ribs flaring out or gripping downward (figure 3.4 and 3.5)?

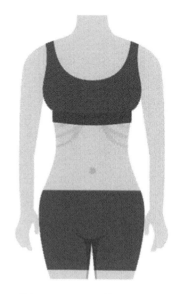

*Figure 3.4: Ribs Flaring*

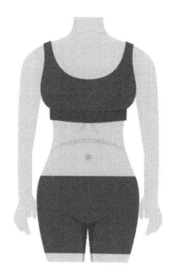

*Figure 3.5: Ribs Gripping*

## Ribs Flaring

You might notice your ribs flaring outward as you try to engage the core. Ribs flaring could be due to poor posture, or you may be using the wrong abdominal muscles. It could also be because of the ribs current positioning, which sometimes alters during a pregnancy.

Your diaphragm sits underneath your rib cage. Think back to the canister analogy we talked about earlier. If the top of the canister is thrusted forward, something will have to give, and it will probably be your back. Imagine if you take a big inhale now, the inhale cannot reach the back easily and it will always be directed forward. If your rib cage is tilted forward, then can you think about the pressure that your diaphragm is sending down as you inhale? It will keep pushing to the front and stress your upper diastasis or above-navel diastasis. Hence the wider angle your ribs are, the more likely you are to have an upper diastasis recti as your ribs are pulling the muscles away from the center.

If so, focus your breathing work above the navel and use a pillow to prop up your head and shoulders while doing your breathing exercises lying supine on the floor. Postural exercises are very important too. We will discuss posture in the next secret.

## Ribs Gripping

Ribs gripping is when you are gripping down the front of your ribs, similar to slouching. You end up rounding your upper back and your shoulders tilt forward in this clenching position. And now if you tuck your bottom, your stomach will look like it is pushing out rather than pulling inward. Think of your core canister being compressed. Your abdomen gets inflated with unnecessary intra-abdominal pressure, creating a bigger belly than usual.

If you continuously grip your ribs while moving and engaging your muscles, then you may be putting a tremendous amount of pressure on the pelvic floor. This can lead to pelvic floor dysfunction.

The reason why you see ribs flaring or gripping is most likely your bad posture, poor alignment and execution during exercises, and/or habitual gripping and holding due to stress and other factors.

We will discover and understand more as we go through this book. First, you need to learn and practice how to engage your TA muscles properly, especially when lying on your back before you can move further. Then you must learn how to engage your TA while standing, sitting and lying on the side, and holding yourself up with proper alignment.

## Three Types of Breathing to Avoid

The three types of ineffective breathing are 1)shallow breathing, 2)belly breathing, and 3) paradoxical breathing.

- **Shallow breathing** is when you are breathing into your chest, shoulder and neck area. You will see that your shoulders are rising up toward your ears. Your chest expands but your belly stays put. In this case, first relax your belly entirely, then take a deep inhale. Your chest should expand along with your belly. Your shoulders should barely move. Try putting your hands on your chest and your belly to feel it.

- **Belly breathing** is the opposite. This is when you see your belly balloon up as you inhale, usually much faster and higher than your chest. There is no muscle expansion on the sides of your ribs and back. Again, practice distributing your inhale equally between your chest, sides and belly.

- **Paradoxical breathing** is when your chest and side of the ribs expands, but your belly sucks inward instead of expanding naturally. In this case, when you inhale, your diaphragm draws upward creating a vacuum effect. Here, you are disrupting the normal breathing pattern.

Master the 360-degree inhale before moving on to the exhale. A deep exhale is as important as a deep inhale. Record yourself so you can replay it for feedback.

I often see moms with severe DR belly breathe, because the core muscle is widely stretched out and the abdomen has little support. Hence, the inhaled breath goes straight to the belly button area.

The cycle of exercising the core to strengthen it and then stressing it with belly breathing all day, will never end. It is a constant tug of war. Think about it, when you exercise, you breathe into your belly. When you rest, you breathe into your belly. How do you expect it to flatten?

Hence, the correct breathing technique is incredibly important, and it comes with a good, deep exhale to activate the TA. This is the biggest change you can make for the most impact.

Without proper deep breathing and activating the transverse abdominal muscles, we won't get very far on our quest. Breathing exercises are your foundation, and it is crucial to your success. I know I'm repeating myself, but I cannot stress enough how important this step is! For some people, this may take a few days or a few weeks. You may feel a little sore, like mild menstrual cramps, or you may not feel like it is doing anything, but trust the process.

**Checklist:**

1. Are you breathing in and out too fast?

2. Is your chest expanding with your belly?

3. Is your back arching when you lie on your back? - you can bolster your head and shoulders with pillows.

4. Are you using your mental awareness and hands to guide you?

5.  Do you see your belly button moving upward or inward when you are standing or sitting?

6.  Can you use a different cue to lift your pelvic floor: bringing a marble up, pretending you are sucking a smoothie, stopping the flow of your urine?

7.  Do you feel any pressure pressing down on your pelvic floor as you inhale? You shouldn't have that feeling. If the symptom persists, stop deep breathing and seek help from your doctor.

## Sucking in your Tummy All Day

It is impossible to suck in your tummy all day, even if you want to. Your body doesn't function like that. You consciously engage the TA, and you might be activating it during that focused period, but as soon as you are distracted, you will let go. Naturally, you don't engage your body that way. Even if you can suck in our tummies all day, and I mean activating the TA muscles here, you shouldn't.

You want to expand and contract the belly, so the muscles get a workout. If you are in the 'flexed' position all the time, it doesn't do anything to the muscles. You are only worsening the muscle which then becomes hypertonic (an overactive muscle).

Next time, when you are brushing your teeth, or sitting down to work or read this book, contract and expand your belly randomly to warm up the muscles. Then, do the TA exercise. The more you do it, the more comfortable you will get with it, and you will be able to activate it on demand throughout the day.

# Chapter 4:

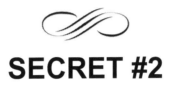

# SECRET #2

## Posture Matters

Posture involves keeping the body straight and upright while performing daily activities such as carrying your baby, pushing the stroller and walking.

Poor posture puts undue stress on your spine as it has become fixed in an abnormal position. This is one of the main reasons why you may be experiencing back pain.

## Posture Awareness

Take a look at yourself while standing sideways in front of the mirror. Do you see yourself leaning forward or backward?

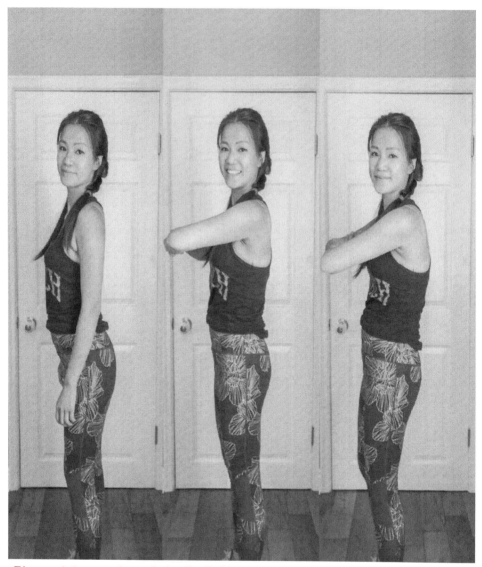

*Figure 4.1: anterior pelvic tilt (left), neutral (middle), posterior pelvic tilt (right)*

Can you tell in which photo I am standing correctly? Pay attention to my butt! The answer is the middle picture. Do you see that I am not sticking my bottom out? I am in a neutral position with a gentle curve in my lower back. I am also lightly engaging my transverse abdominal muscles.

My posture on the left is called the anterior pelvic tilt, when your bottom is sticking out. You generally have a high arch on your back stiffening your back muscles. You have tight hamstrings and are not very flexible. Your ribs may flare out, misaligned with the position of your pelvis; think of a bent canister.

The right side of the picture is called the posterior pelvic tilt. You clench your bottom, sometimes unconsciously. You are generally slouchier, and you hunch forward. Your shoulders are rounded and misaligned with your ears and your upper back is stiff; think of a squashed canister.

One of the biggest postpartum posture issues is the misalignment of your hips. For nine months you walked around with a rapidly changing body, adjusting your posture to stay balanced. So, you need to teach your body how to re-align. Sometimes, you sway forward as if you still have a baby inside your tummy, and you arch your spines. This can increase the chances of arthritis because the joints connecting to the spine are constantly strained. You also hang on to the fascial support in the front of your core instead of it being aligned. On the top, your rib cage is shifted forward, which doesn't allow you to take the good 360-degree breathing we mentioned in secret #1. Your ribcage needs to be aligned in such a way that allows your breath to go down to your pelvic floor.

The middle picture finds the middle ground between the two postures, and you should aim for this alignment because it will allow you to fully support your spine. Check for the following:

1. Shoulders underneath your ears.

2. Ribs stacked above the hips.

3. Hips not sticking way out nor tucked under.

4. Neutral curve in the back.

5. Knees are soft so your quad muscles can relax slightly.

6. Weight is evenly balanced between your heels and the ball of your feet.

## How to Correct Your Posture

Now, take a picture with your phone of your side view while standing, like the one above. With this image, we can analyze your posture together. It's best to have someone take it for you.

Pay attention to the alignment on your photo: 1) head 2) shoulders 3) ribs and 4) hips.

What do you see?

Be aware of the areas we talked about above, and circle the problem areas in your photo.

Here are some general rules and tips that you need for optimal function so you can be strong and feel great:

1. Chest up but keep the ribcage down so it doesn't flare out. Keeping the ribcage down means repositioning the upper part of your body.

2. Stand tall but not military tall, so your shoulders are relaxed.

3. Ribcage is stacked horizontally above your pelvis, keeping them connected. (figure 4.1 neutral)

4. Tilt your pelvis forward or backward slightly. The arch on your back should not be excessive nor submissive. Find a neutral curve on the back and align your pelvis with your ribcage as #3.

5. Body weight should be evenly distributed on both hips.

6. Supportive footwear should be worn when standing for prolonged period.

7. Your knees should not be locked.

8. Engage your TA lightly.

9. Pretend that a string is pulling you up like a puppet, so your neck is long.

10. Stretch your hip flexors and hamstrings

Are you putting more weight on one foot than the other? Are you constantly looking down on your phone? Do you have uneven shoulders? If so, working on the weaker side (normally the lower shoulder) will help.

I am squarely guilty of bad posture, especially in the beginning of my journey. I slouched too much because I felt awkward when I stood tall or I'd throw my shoulders back since I hadn't been standing that way forever. But once I became more mindful of my posture, it became more natural. It's not too late to correct your posture, but you need to start now.

The goal here is to set new standards and self-monitor frequently. I understand it is hard to change our posture overnight. Try setting many alarms on your phone or smartwatch throughout the day to remind yourself to sit, stand and walk in good alignment. While you are healing and strengthening your core, your posture will become better too. This is the beauty of the human body: it's all cogs and wheels. When you work on one part of your body, the other parts of the body will start working with you.

In secret #5, I will show you how stretches will help with your diastasis and help you realign your body. It's important to note that posture isn't just about standing, yoga poses or sitting straight. Finding a new neutral alignment, as opposed to your existing dominant posture, will help you use your core more effectively especially when you exercise. You will breathe better, reduce your back pain, and prevent you from injury.

## Your Everyday Movements

Your everyday movements can all add up to helping support better posture. Try be mindful of the following things during everyday tasks:

1. Don't hunch over to pick up stuff from the floor. Often, you casually bend down to the floor to pick something up, but this can put a lot of stress on your back. Instead, bend your knees in a slight squat, engage your core, then grab what you need off the floor.

2. Picking up a toddler or something heavy. Instead of hunching over and lifting her, place one knee on the floor, the other knee bent at 90 degrees. Place your toddler on that leg, and engage your TA as you lift her.

3. Going from a lying position to a seated position. Always roll onto your side and push yourself up with your arms.

4. Going from a sitting position to lying on the back. Use your arms to lower yourself from a seated position to a side-lying

position first; then, once your head and shoulder touches the bed or the floor, you can roll onto your back, and always engage your TA while rolling around.

5. Be aware of your posture when you push the stroller. Can you adjust the handle, so you are not slouching forward?

6. Is your breastfeeding position optimal for your core? Are your shoulders relaxed and your arms well supported? Use a feeding pillow and bring the baby towards yourself instead of leaning forward.

7. When you bring your arms up to shampoo your hair, are you arching your back and flaring out the ribs? Try to keep your alignment in place even while washing your hair.

8. Holding your baby. Are you putting her on top of your belly pooch as a cushion? This position will make your upper back tilt backwards. Imagine your linea alba is a zipper. If you bend backwards without activating your TA, it would break the zipper and force it open (okay, maybe not to that extreme!). On the other hand, are you sticking your hip out to one side and have your baby clamming on to your side, so the other side of your ribs flare out? That's also not good for your posture. If you need to carry your baby for long stretches, then I suggest using a carrier that has excellent back support.

Not only will you have a better posture, but you will also have a pair of free hands!

It takes a great deal of practice and mindfulness to hold yourself up. In fact, you burn calories just by standing with good posture! Think about your lifestyle and use every opportunity you have to utilize your muscle structure to hold yourself up, so you can recruit your abs as much as you can. This is your natural alignment, so you'll feel great about doing your daily tasks instead of constantly stressing your back or abs. Make it fun, and you are going to have an easier time healing your diastasis.

# Chapter 5:

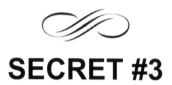

# SECRET #3

## A Belly Wrap

If you've understood everything I have revealed so far, then you are off to a great start! Now here is a little-known secret that makes a big difference – wearing a bottom-up belly wrap.

## Belly Wrap Myths

You have been told that:

- A belly wrap will put pressure on your pelvic floor.

- A belly wrap will decrease your muscle memory.

- A belly wrap is restrictive, and it decreases your blood flow.

IT'S NOT TRUE!

If you are wearing the right belly wrap in the right way, then it will speed up your postpartum recovery and help heal your DR.

## Explore the Different Types of Belly Wrap

As the name suggests, it's a product you wrap around your waist to support your body. A postpartum belly wrap is designed to be worn shortly after giving birth, so the mother is warmed, can move around with better support against gravity, and get back to pre-baby shape quicker.

Before I wore the belly wrap, there was no muscle contraction in my tummy, and I felt that everything inside the abdominal area was wobbling at every step I took. When I wore my wrap, I instantly felt that my guts were held securely in place, and my back was supported. I could maneuver better with my daily tasks.

For example, when I bent down to grab a toy off the floor, the light compression from the wrap would hold my stomach in place from the pull of gravity. So, it reminded me to bend properly and engage the tummy.

The belly wrap instantly made me look better with a less protruding stomach- This is a cosmetic perk!

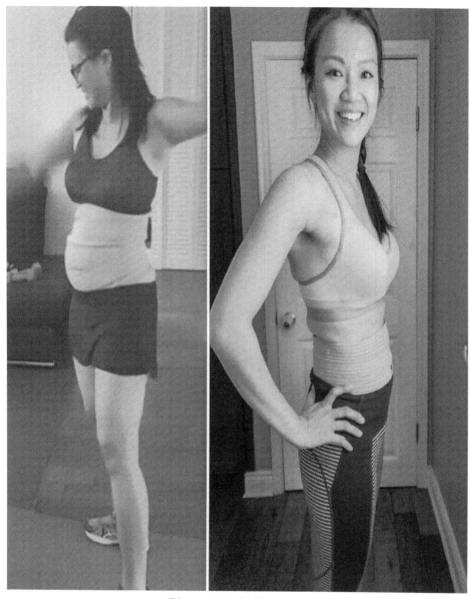

*Figure 5.1: belly wrap*

Most importantly, wearing the wrap sped up the recovery of my diastasis recti, especially in the beginning. I remember going back to see my physiotherapist for my follow up appointment two weeks after the first visit. I had no idea if I'd made any improvement. But when she told me that I'd closed one finger gap, I was pleasantly surprised!

I find that having a proper belly wrap helps:

1. Support the pelvis and the overly stretched tissues in the abdominal wall.

2. Guide diastasis recti moms into restorative posture and alignment.

3. Provide support, warmth and light compression through daily activities.

4. Protect the core during high intra-abdominal pressure events such as sneezing and coughing.

Postpartum belly wrapping is a tradition in many countries such as China, Japan, Mexico, Brazil, India, Malaysia and Indonesia. And many celebrities rely on it too to get back into shape quickly.

According to a study published in Physiotherapy Canada, postpartum wrapping may help women get back on their feet sooner and walk farther. It may also help women have less pain, distress and bleeding after a C-section, according to a second study published in the International Journal of Gynaecology and Obstetrics.

One way to wrap your tummy, as is done in many traditional cultures, is to use a long running piece of soft breathable fabric, and start wrapping yourself from around your underwear line and slowly moving up and covering your entire belly. There are several videos online that teach you different methods of doing this yourself. This is a very comfortable and safe wrap, but it can be time consuming to tie the wrap and is effective only if you get the right amount of compression.

There are a lot of ready-made wraps available in the market too. However, not every postpartum wrap is created the same. Some are recommended by doctors and physios, and some are not. A lot of products out there claim to help you get in shape, and make you look good cosmetically when worn underneath clothes. But you want to be extra careful when it comes to choosing a wrap suitable to diastasis recti because we need to make sure it provides the support you need, and not unnecessary pressure like squeezing the middle of your stomach.

Let's explore the different types of belly binders on the market.

# Corset

A corset is mostly a shaping garment. It is to be worn underneath your clothes, so you will appear to have a fuller bust and flatter stomach. It is usually made out of slightly stretchy fabric with the closure made of many metal hooks. Some of them require you to hook around the crotch area. A corset is not suitable for those with DR. I can only imagine how confining it would be with all the hooks in the middle and the bottom.

## Waist Trainer

Waist Trainers are wide, adjustable bands that cover the middle of your midsection. You will most commonly see it in the gym, on celebrity trainers and personal trainers. They are often made of stiffer materials and may contain plastic and metal boning. Their purpose is to put firm compression on the waist so the user sweats more and sucks in the abs more. This too is not suitable for those with DR.

## High Waist Shaper Undergarment

A high waist shaper undergarment is designed to be worn as an underwear to help lift your butt, and shape your tummy. It is usually made of nylon, and some have wires in them to provide extra firmness. The shaper underwear is a quickie. You will commonly find women wearing this type of undergarment, especially when they are wearing a tight fitted dress or top. It is suitable if your diastasis recti is mild or moderate.

## Belly Wrap or Belly Binder

A belly binder is generally a wide, adjustable and stretchable velcro band that covers your abdomen from your ribs down to the tops of your hips. It is similar to a waist trainer, but it provides compression on a larger area. You tighten it with a velcro strap. This is what we will explore.

You may commonly see this type of binder (figure 5.2), which is a wide wrap with two stretchable velcro straps on either side to secure and tighten it. I used to wear this wrap but I quickly realized how uncomfortable it was. If you have a massive belly like I did, THIS WON'T WORK.

Imagine if you are trying to wrap a present, and the present is a balloon. How are you supposed to wrap a balloon neatly with paper? You cannot wrap it seamlessly without leaving pockets of air.

The same is true with the above belly binder; it needs to hug and evenly support your entire belly, not putting all the pressure in the middle of your stomach. Can you imagine where all the pressure goes? This type of wrap will put downward pressure on your tummy which can cause issues in your pelvic floor. It can also cause the pressure to go upward which messes up your diaphragm which messes up your deep breathing.

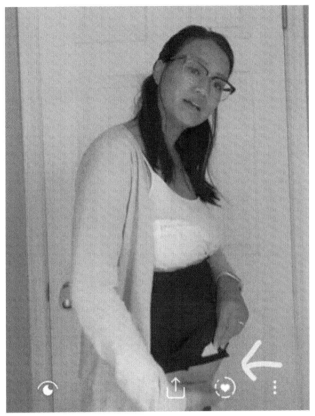

*Figure 5.2: commonly found belly wrap in the market. Poor engineer for moms with a huge belly.*

## DR-Friendly Belly Wrap

A good DR-friendly belly wrap should be a stretchable wrap with several straps that can spread throughout your abdomen area to create a hugging effect. It is made to wrap your belly starting from the underwear line and up to your rib cage. You want a wrap that is suitable for your size, not one fabric that fits all. The belly wrap should be hugging your belly snugly so it doesn't leave gaps at the top and the bottom of your tummy.

Since it is wrapping from the bottom up and it has multiple straps, it would not rise or move easily. Imagine when you sit down on a chair, the straps will spread evenly, whereas the one-piece would have nowhere to go except for rising up and digging into your chest.

The right belly wrap should be able to:

1. Compliment your fitness exercises.

2. Provide 360-degree security, and protect your belly and your back from being pulled on by gravity.

3. Provide moderate compression that reminds you to engage the TA and have a better posture.

4. Support the pelvis and the tissues in the abdominal wall.

5. Decrease pressure on your back. As you can imagine the mom pooch carries some weight in the front which your back compensates for.

6. Keep you warm, which will increase your blood flow and speed up the recovery.

7. Provide overall comfort and support.

8. Cosmetically looks good under clothes, and it temporarily makes your belly flatter after you take off the wrap, see picture below. (Ultimately, you need to exercise and eat right for a sustainable result.)

As you can see, there are a lot of benefits from wearing a diastasis-friendly belly wrap.

## When to Wear a Belly Wrap

If you have severe DR (beginner stage), I would recommend wearing it twenty-four hours a day, except when you shower, for at least six weeks. Wash it as often as you need to since you will exercise in it.

If you have a moderate DR (intermediate stage), you may wear it during your workout and throughout the day. Then take it off from time to time to see how your linea alba responds in terms of your movements and core tension, especially when you're trying a new exercise. You need to know that you can handle the specific exercises, but if you're recording yourself and the wrap blocks your view of your body, it will also block your judgment.

If you are advanced, you do not need to wear one.

It's important to note that it doesn't matter whether you are 2 weeks, 6 months or a year postpartum, if you are in the beginner stage of trying to recover your diastasis, wearing a belly wrap will help you achieve the result faster.

We will talk about DR stages when we talk about exercises.

## When Not to Wear a Belly Wrap

While belly binding can undoubtedly help give support while you are wearing it, it doesn't fix the problem in the long run.

Your core is somewhat protected while using the belly wrap, and this is beneficial, especially for moms with moderate to severe diastasis recti. But at some point, you want to make the core muscles do their job. And that is by having the core fully relaxed before drawing in the navel. The broader distance of the pulling motion will make the muscle work much harder.

To achieve long-term gain and to heal holistically, you must look at strengthening the core from the inside out. It starts with 360-degree breathing and engaging your transverse abdominal muscles in a good posture. You can then progressively load the core with more exercises, then with a high-intensity total body workout, and nourish your core. You will discover the details in the rest of this book.

# Chapter 6:

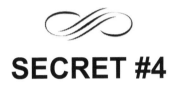

# SECRET #4

## Tension

Can I do yoga?

Can I do Pilates?

Can I run?

Can I swim?

Can I do CrossFit?

Can I lift weights?

Can I (fill in the blank)?

# What Exercise Can I Do?

Instead of asking, 'Can I do yoga?', you should ask, 'Is this exercise suitable for this stage of my DR journey?' Anyone can do yoga, but should you do it at this moment? You need to understand whether you can generate enough tension in your linea alba, which is the vertical mid-section of your tummy where you see doming or bulging with DR.

## Tension and The Gap

When you search the internet, diastasis recti is commonly measured by a finger-width gap or in centimeters, indicating how severe the DR is. That's why many people think that if they can close the gap, then they will heal the diastasis recti.

While this is true, when you close the gap, it signifies that the external core is back to how it should be. However, if your gap is not closed, it does not mean that you won't get a strong core, or the flat belly you ultimately want. You need to pay attention to the function in your core.

Most people commonly neglect the tension in their linea alba. The linea alba is a fibrous connective tissue made mostly of collagen, that runs down the midline of the abdomen. It is the thin white sheet (figure 2.1) that holds the core muscles together.

Imagine your tummy is a volleyball net (figure 6.1). The net itself is the linea alba. You want to move the poles (TA) on either side so that the net is not loose. When your linea alba is strong and taut, it can withstand intra-abdominal pressure while you switch positions, exercise and cough.

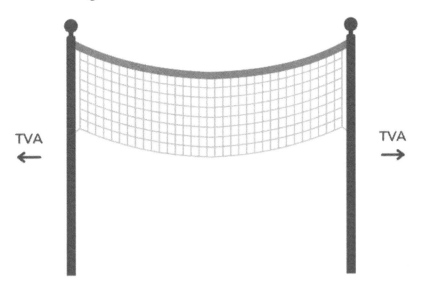

TVA ←

TVA →

*Figure 6.1: Imagining the linea alba is the net*

## Feeling the Linea Alba

1. Lie on your back, engage your TA muscles, lift your head off the floor, and point your chin towards the chest.

2. Put your fingers along the midline of your abdomen and gently press your linea alba. Can you feel any tension or firmness in the linea alba when you are engaging your core?

If it is soft, how many fingers can you fit in and how deep does it go?

If you were to throw a dime into the linea alba area, would it sink in, or would it bounce off like it would off your cheeks? You may notice that there is more tension in some positions than others. Every now and then, you want to feel the intensity in various positions to see if there is any improvement. You will find yourself holding steadier in one position than the other.

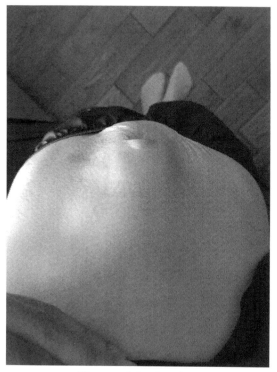

*Figure 6.2: doming*

Do you see the doming, gap sinking or bulging on your stomach while you exercise, lift your child or get up from the bed? This indicates poor tension in the linea alba.

Gap sinking is the opposite of doming in which you will see your gap becomes hollow as you can sink your fingers in. Bulging is when you see your stomach bunch up and bulges forming a round circular shape. The bulge is filled with intra-abdominal pressure, so when you touch the bulging area, it could feel hardened.

This photo (figure 6.2) was taken when I leaned my upper back backward while standing up.

In all cases above, they are due to the lack of strength in your core muscles, mainly the transverse abdominal muscle, think of the volleyball net in figure 6.1.

# Recognizing the Current Stage of Your DR Journey

## 1. Beginner Stage

At this stage, you might be a new mom, or months or years postpartum, with moderate to severe diastasis measurements. You've only just found out that you have diastasis recti, you don't know where or how to start, or you've tried a few things but without any results. You always see doming and bulging whenever you are moving around. You might be in pain. You have weight to lose, and you are not very active.

## 2. Intermediate Stage

At this stage, you have learned how to engage your deep core muscle and breathe properly. You have been engaging your TA for a while now, and you feel that you can activate it on demand. You have tried different types of diastasis exercises, and you may have tried some mid to low impact workouts. You are somewhat active, but the mommy pooch is still there, and doming is visible.

### A Mix of Beginner and Intermediate

This is where you might have one technique but not the other. For example, you are somewhat active, you have been activating your TA, but you are not aware that you are a shallow breather for example.

## 3. Advanced Stage

You have tried everything. You are able to breathe 360-degree throughout your exercises, you have a good posture, and you can engage your TA well while maintaining proper tension in the linea alba through different exercises. You are doing mid to high impact exercises consistently. You might have lost all the baby weight, but your tummy has plateaued, and it won't go away. You can't figure out why.

## What Do the Stages Mean to You?

It means that you should not compare yourself with others because we are all at different stages of our journey. Those exercises you find online might be too easy for you. Or you might not yet be ready to handle what is recommended in a cookie cutter DR program.

What I have found from my experience and research is that most people make diastasis recti scarier than it is. 'You shouldn't do this!' 'You should always avoid that!' 'This exercise will 100 percent worsen your gap.'

We are always in this fearful mindset because of all the mixed messages out there. You have to stop being scared of causing damage to your separation because you are not going to force it, and I am going to teach you how.

You need to shift the focus from avoidance to recognizing where you are at, determine what you can and cannot handle, and then challenge yourself to progress. This is probably the most important thing I can teach you in this book. Because if you are only doing leg slides, pelvic tilts, dead bug etc. and wondering why you are not getting the flat belly, then your understanding of your condition is incomplete.

## Targeted Diastasis Recti Exercises

Having said that, here is a general list of specifically targeted diastasis exercises for the three different stages. But I don't want you to think that you need to keep repeating these moves forever. These exercises will become your DR modifications as we move on to talk about why you need a high-intensity total body workout later.

Note for new moms: your body needs time to heal and get back into running shape. Take care of yourself and be gentle. Wait for your doctor's go ahead before you start any exercise routine. And when you do, if you are ever in doubt about an activity, ask your doctor. They can help assess how you are doing and whether you are ready for more strenuous activity.

## Beginner Stage Exercise

Walking is essential, especially if you are a new mom. Practice activating your TA as you walk, and make it your goal to walk 10,000 steps a day. If you are walking with a stroller, be sure you are not slouching forward. DR workout typically includes breathing exercises, postural exercises, knee lift, heel slide, pelvic tilt, glute bridge, heel tap, wall plank, clam, and mini squat. You will focus heavily on breathing and activating the TA muscles in various positions mentioned in secret #1.

## Intermediate Stage Exercise

You should be able to go on your hands and knees in a table top position while engaging your TA. When you feel comfortable, you can do squats, lunges, palloff presses, modified bird dog, modified dead bug, modified plank on a table or the wall, modified side plank with one knee on the floor. Mainly modifications of the advanced exercises. For example, instead of lifting your leg up and out, you would simply slide the leg out. Instead of a traditional dead bug, bend your knee and tap the floor.

## Advanced Stage Exercise

At this stage, you have progressively monitored your body's reactions and are able to add more resistance to challenge your core. Exercises include one leg extension and lift, scissors, mini crunch, full dead bug, c-curve and hold, boat, floor plank, double legs lift, side plank, hundred in Pilates, and palloff presses with heavier resistance bands.

**Remember -** When you do any of these diastasis recti exercises, you are breathing, engaging your TA muscles and holding yourself with proper alignment as you do them. For example, for a knee lift, as you lift your knee, you are inhaling when you are relaxed and not exerting energy, and when you move, you exhale and engage the TA. When you do a dead bug, each time you are extending your arm and leg, you are exhaling and engaging the TA.

You are probably surprised that I mention crunches and planks because they seem like such a diastasis curse! Isn't it well known that these will worsen your diastasis gap?

THEY WON'T!

As your core gets stronger, your linea alba tension will improve. Therefore, you will be able to withstand the pressure from a crunch. Also, because you are now in the advanced stage, you need to start building your external core muscles so it can hold everything in place and get you a stronger core.

It's crucial that you get equal strength among all four layers of core muscles. The external core (upper abs and the lower abs or recti abdominis also known as the six-pack muscles), external and internal obliques, and your deep core (TA); otherwise, your belly could look disproportionate like a bread loaf.

Keep in mind, our goal here is for you to understand what stage of the diastasis journey you are in, and become familiar with targeted DR exercises that activate your TA muscles.

## Two Important Questions

Two questions you want to ask yourself when you are doing the diastasis recti exercises:

1. Is this too easy for my core?

2. Is this too hard for my core?

Most often than not, you misinterpret the technique on 360-degree breathing and engaging your TA, or you're doing exercises that are too easy and without enough variety. For example, you always lift weights, and you diligently lift them four times a week, month after month. You are lifting the exact same weight, doing the same repetition, of course, your body is not going to change dramatically because your body has adapted to it, it becomes too easy. Why bother?

If you are looking to maintain, and are wildly happy with your strength and appearance, then that's great! But if you are reading this book, then it's likely that you want to look better, especially on the tummy, right? Then you need to challenge your muscles; it's a principle called 'progressive overload'.

According to the American College of Sports Medicine's Resources for the Personal Trainer fifth edition, "To improve muscular fitness, the muscles must be exposed to an overload (stress beyond typical activity). This is done via resistance training. Over time, as the muscles adapt to a given overload, the training stimulus must be increased to continue to have gains. This is referred to as **progressive overload."**

In other words, it forces your muscles to do more by adding a little more intensity at a time.

Nothing will change unless you challenge yourself, and this principle can be applied to life and also to our human body. If you stay in your comfort zone, how far will you go? The principle of progressive overload is essential to getting desired results. You will find it easy to overload your muscles when you follow Secret #5. As a matter of fact, all the secrets I have revealed so far ARE golden keys to your flat belly, but you must follow them in sequence. You cannot skip ahead to DR exercises without knowing how to engage your TA.

Do you get it? You have to let go of your fear that the exercises are going to worsen your gap. Instead, learn to judge whether the activity is too hard or too easy for you at this point.

## Indication of an Exercise Being Too Hard

Remember, after I gave birth to my first baby, I jumped straight into a high-intensity full-body workout program without knowing that I had diastasis recti. I didn't know how to engage my core correctly and pushed myself too much. I thought if I can lose all my excess weight, my belly would go too. I know a lot of women who felt the same way too. No one ever told us what diastasis recti was. Since I didn't have the correct form or a proper technique in breathing and engaging my TA, the workout was too difficult for my core.

## The Secret 'Too Hard' Indicator

The most important indicator of an exercise being too hard is the linea alba doming and bulging – the 'mountain' that forms in the abdomen or the round bulge that is hardened on your belly. You may also see sinking, as if your belly button disappears into the gap, or you may feel yourself bearing down, which is forcing too much pressure down to your pelvic floor as if you are having a hard time in the bathroom.

Keep in mind that every movement has the potential to raise the intra-abdominal pressure (figure 6.3). What is important to note is whether we have bad control, good control or great control of it. Munira mentions that "doming and bulging didn't cause the pressure. It is a window into seeing what's happening inside the abdomen and how the muscles and tissues are responding to it.

Use it as feedback to assess your ability to control it." In other words, you want to be able to manage and contain the core pressure as you exercise. The amount of core pressure is different for every exercise. Hence, the harder and more front loaded an exercise is, the more pressure you need to manage, and the harder it is for your core. After she said that, it made so much sense to me. When I first started doing planks on the floor, I was hesitant as I could feel a little bit of doming. However, I was not bulging and I wasn't struggling to maintain my alignment, so I knew it was okay for me to do.

When you are doing Pilates, check your core. How is your tension?
Is it great control, good control or bad control (figure 6.3) ?

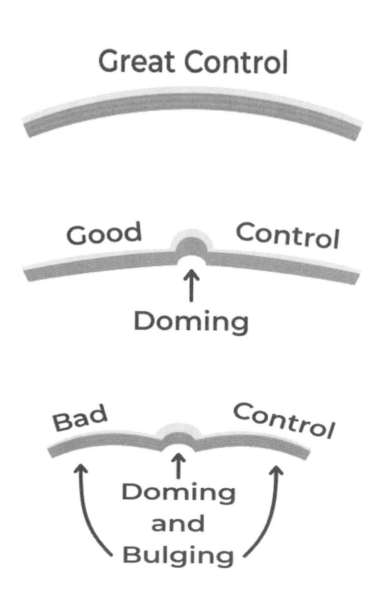

*Figure 6.3: great control, good control or bad control. Your control of the intra-abdominal pressure while doing any exercise*

When you are spinning, how is your control in the first five minutes? How about fifteen minutes later?

Do you have great control when you do the first few reps of the exercise?

As you do a few more, your core muscles may become fatigued, and you might struggle to maintain the tension and start bearing down. You may go from having great control to bad control. In this case, decrease the intensity or shorten the duration. Take a short break, then take a deep 360-degree inhale, and re-engage your TA before trying it again. You also want to make sure that you do your exercises in the correct form from beginning to end.

If you are running or doing a high impact activity, pay attention to if there's any pressure on your pelvic floor. We will discuss the pelvic floor in detail in section 3.

So next time, while you are in Zen, look at yourself in the mirror and ask: Can I maintain the linea alba tension doing this warrior pose, and how long can I maintain it for? Can I do the downward dog without compromising the pressure? Can I lift the dumbbells with a proper posture and maintain great tension? Can I feel trembling in my core ? If you can control your tension with a little bit of doming, but can maintain it for a few breaths, that's okay!

Recognizing where you are in your diastasis journey is imperative. I often feel that some women with DR can handle many activities they like, such as running, yoga, or modified normal ab exercises, but they are afraid to try. Don't be scared to practice the more advanced moves because your body will let you know whether you are ready for it.

## Track Your Tension

Take some time now and track your tension. Our goal is to feel firmness when engaging the TA muscles, which is important as we move on to the exercises. I have created two charts for you, so you can track your before and after linea alba tension.

Check your tension now and write it down in the tracker.

# Linea Alba Tension Tracker

1. Activate your TA, circle the firmness of the Linea Alba from 1 to 4.
2. 1- Softest ( A coin can sink in), 4 (a coin will bounce off)

**Before/ Date:**

| | | | | |
|---|---|---|---|---|
| Lie Down | 1 | 2 | 3 | 4 |
| Sit Down | 1 | 2 | 3 | 4 |
| Stand Up | 1 | 2 | 3 | 4 |

**After/ Date:**

| | | | | |
|---|---|---|---|---|
| Lie Down | 1 | 2 | 3 | 4 |
| Sit Down | 1 | 2 | 3 | 4 |
| Stand Up | 1 | 2 | 3 | 4 |

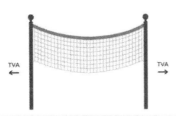

# Chapter 7:

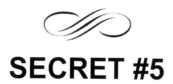

# SECRET #5

## A High-Intensity Total Body Workout

When my physio told me that I had to lie on the floor and engage my core with my breath and do nothing else for the first six weeks, I fell asleep almost every time I exercised. Imagine a tired, sleep-deprived mom, busy with her toddler and baby and work all day, and you ask her to lie down and just breathe? You'd rather just ask her to take a nap. Plus, how often can you lie down by yourself without getting interrupted and being crawled over? #momlife right?

I do not enjoy monotonous static repetition too much. However, those breathing exercises are your foundation and building blocks.

The key is to get the hang of the basics and then incorporate them into progressively intense workouts, while having fun.

After giving birth to my daughter Emily in May 2018, I'd gained over 25 lbs again. I felt terrible with my body image. I thought to myself, "Is this how I am supposed to look now that I'm a mom? Maybe this is how it's supposed to be ... my metabolism is slower now ... just wear something baggy."

But deep down, I refused to buy a brand-new wardrobe of clothes. I only wore maternity clothes, and I would purposely buy boring clothes, so I could become more motivated to lose weight and get rid of the belly.

At that time, I was taking care of Emily and her brother, and they kept me on my toes all the time. How many times do you say, "my exercise is carrying my baby up and down the stairs all day"? How many times do you say, "chasing after my kids is my cardio"? I told myself this stuff all the time, but I realized these were excuses.

I didn't see my body change after chasing around my kids or walking the stairs. I was so frustrated. Then, I remembered doing this high-intensity full-body workout after I had Jordan, which helped me lose 20 lbs by working out on my own time and at home. I knew I could do it again!

What if I combined secrets #1 to #4 into the full-body workout? Wouldn't I be able to lose weight and heal my DR at the same time?

In August 2018, I started to substitute anything I could not handle with the targeted DR exercises mentioned in secret #4.

I made sure I engaged the TA throughout the movement properly while having my belly wrapped. And I also followed secret #6, which we'll discuss later. It was so much fun, and I was motivated to do the exercise!

As you can see in the following picture (figure 7.1), the results were terrific after just one month. I knew this approach worked. I was able to exercise at home, on my schedule, with no one staring at me except for my kids, haha!

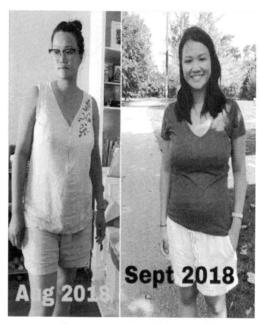

*Figure 7.1: one month progression, I lost 7 lbs and a few inches.*

I continued to tweak and modified so that the workout was suitable for the severe type of diastasis. While gaining new knowledge through research and courses, I incorporated what I learnt, experimented and corrected the mistake I made that may have stressed the core. It truly has been a tried and tested method, you never knew until you tried! And this was how the Tummy Warrior Method was born!

## Why You Need to Work Your Entire Body to Heal Diastasis Recti

It is a proven fact that exercises enhance a person's overall health when done on a regular basis. What's more important is that your body needs a variety of exercises hitting each area so you can build lean muscle, increase your metabolism, and burn fat all day. By combining the five elements below with emphasis on engaging your TA, 360-degree breathing, and alignment, you will prevent training plateaus. And it will also help you to avoid burnout and weariness since you won't be doing the same routine every day. Most importantly, with this approach you will be progressively overloading your muscles which is exactly what you need as you recall from secret #4. The variety of exercises in different planes and range of motion, slow and fast, will generate a contrasting intra-abdominal pressure to challenge your core. Every exercise becomes your core exercise. This is the magic to lose weight and heal your diastasis recti at the same time.

In addition, our mid-section usually carries extra fat from the pregnancy. If you are doing the DR exercises alone, then they are not going to help you lose weight and melt the fat away. Your core may strengthen, but your mummy tummy will look the same. This is one of the main reasons why moms complain that their bellies show no sign of flattening, despite them doing their DR core work diligently. DR exercises alone won't help you get a flat stomach.

A high-intensity total body workout combines five elements:

1. high-intensity interval training (HIIT),

2. strength training,

3. core exercises,

4. balance training, and

5. flexibility and stretching.

These five elements practiced together is what I call "Progressive Combo Training" in my Tummy Warrior Method.

But don't confuse a high-intensity workout with a high-impact workout. High-intensity means that you are doing the exercise to your maximum ability within a period at your own pace, usually forty to sixty seconds, then followed by a rest period or a medium-intensity exercise set. And then you will continue to do another set of high-intensity exercise.

It is supposed to keep your heart rate up and make you sweat; however, it does not mean that you have to jump, do burpees or climb mountains like you would with a high-impact workout. If you can't run yet, walk. If you can't jump, then toe-lift. If you can't squat fully, then go as deep as you can. You are challenging yourself to the maximum capacity that you can handle during the interval. Only compare yourself to yesterday's you.

This training is essential. It may sound daunting to someone who hasn't worked out before, and at first, I thought this was nuts too! When I started, I could barely lift my legs off the ground, and at every interval, I ran out of breath at ten seconds already. I had to pause and go back in and pause again. But because it was fast-paced, and I was so focused on the trainer, the workout was finished before I knew it.

Then the next day, I tried again, and again. I noticed I was getting stronger, and I had more energy.

You are going to start where it is appropriate for your core and your fitness level. As you work out, you will gradually build up your strength, and you will have more tolerance in your linea alba tension. These are good signs for your core. And if you are wondering if a particular move is too hard for you, go back to secret

#4 - Tension. Be sure to wear your belly wrap while exercising if you are a beginner.

# Five Elements of Progressive Training to Improve Your Diastasis Recti

## 1. High-Intensity Interval Training (HIIT)

HIIT stimulates the fat burning mechanism in our bodies, and increases your metabolism. Even after you are done working out, you are still burning fat while washing the dishes! Metabolism is a huge factor in weight loss and fat burning. Interval training can be performed through cardio, bodyweight or weightlifting. You will work your entire core while challenging other parts of your body at the same time. You will modify anything you cannot handle with a targeted DR exercise appropriate for your stage within the interval.

## 2. Strength Training

Does lifting weights make DR worse? I hope by now, you are not asking this question anymore! Increased strength allows you to lift heavier objects, and this translates into your personal life on many levels such as lifting the baby's car seat, carrying your toddler, moving the stroller in and out of your car. Simply said, you need power! We all turn into super moms at one point.

When you think of lifting weights, you might be thinking of those gigantic dumbbells! No, silly, start where it is appropriate for you. I started with only water bottles in the beginning and used my daughter as a weight!

Everyone's belly is flatter when it's flexed. When your muscles are weak as with diastasis recti, they won't retain as much tension, so your stomach will distend much more when not flexed. Strength training will help you tone and make you stronger. When you have more lean muscle, you are going to burn fat, and you will look better overall!

## 3. Core Exercises

Remember, it's important that you get equal strength in all four layers of your core muscles. Otherwise, stronger core muscles will take over and do more work instead of your TA muscle, and your belly could appear worse than before.

The reason why two women with the same gap and same depth of diastasis, but their bellies look completely different from each other, is because of the abdominal muscle integrity. Remember, it's natural for the entire abdominal wall to be stretched during pregnancy. For some women, their fascia and muscles are more stretched out than the other women due to hormones, poor shape prior and during pregnancy, inaccurate execution of exercises, a high body mass index (BMI), and how distended the abdomen was (multiple babies, bigger babies, birth after due date).

Therefore, you must not neglect or be shy away from doing normal ab workouts, so you can restore the core normal integrity, or at least, as close as possible. If you are in the beginner stage, you want to start with building the TA muscles, and then work on the internal and external oblique and the six-pack muscles. Core exercises will specifically target those layers.

## 4. Balance Training

In order for optimal movement to occur, your body requires the brain to process sensory information: visual and proprioception (which is the way we perceive our body's position), and vestibular (which is a sense of balance).

In the beginning, you may have no clue that you are doing a particular exercise completely wrong. But after ample practice, it becomes second nature for you to ride a bike, skate, do a tree pose or balance yourself on a yoga ball.

Stability training is great for your core because you need a strong core to have a steady balance. Having good balance will prevent you from falling, and it will also help you to become more agile (the ability to control the direction of your body during movement).

## 5. Flexibility and Stretching

Because of pregnancy, your glutes inevitably become weak. You may arch your back to support the growing belly. You may experience muscle imbalance, which is the incorrect use of underactive and overactive muscles. You may lose your pre-baby level of flexibility. It is also common to have tight hip flexor muscles, ribs flare, and lower back pain due to childbearing.

Hence, you need to focus on realigning your body with stretching and flexibility on a regular basis to realign the skeletal structure that has been adapted to poor posture and exercise habits. Once you develop strength and flexibility in your body, you'll be able to withstand more physical stress, such as carrying your baby, working out, or going about your daily chores. You will have fewer injuries from exercises. It will also help you with muscle imbalances in your body as you will be able to move through a full range of motion, open up the hip flexors, and ultimately, feel less stiff.

Stretching will help release your muscle soreness so you can come back stronger the next day. These exercises go hand-in-hand with good posture discovered in secret #2. Proper alignment and releasing tight hip flexors and hamstrings will make a significant impact on your diastasis recovery.

# Five Tips for Choosing a Program

Take a test drive on their trial membership, and see if you like the program. Consider the following five things before committing to the program:

1. Are the instructions clear and step-by-step? Are there suggested modifications? Can you adapt and apply it to yourself?

2. Does it make you want to do it again or is it boring and makes you dread going back to press play on the computer?

3. Are the workouts varied, rotating the five components or are you repeating the same routine every week?

4. Are there stand-alone demo videos that you repeat on a circuit, or are there work along videos where you are working out with the trainer online/in person? What style do you like?

5. Most importantly, does the program come with a coach or a trainer that will help you look at your alignment and form to see if you are doing the exercise correctly? This is one of the most overlooked factors in healing the core. Correct execution of the exercise is very helpful especially at the beginning stage, so you can have confidence you are doing the exercise correctly and know what to look for based on your core strength and weakness. This will help you save time and money, as well as ensure you gain results a lot quicker.

Time is precious. Let's say your DR exercises take you fifteen minutes every day. Now if you add an extra ten to fifteen minutes of the other fitness elements and have a fun and energetic workout that will help you lose weight, tone and heal the diastasis gap, isn't this a good choice?

## For those with No Extra Weight to Lose

You might be wondering, "what if I have no extra weight to lose?" Would the high-intensity total body workout still be necessary to heal diastasis recti? No, it is not necessary; however, doing only core exercise is not an effective nor a complete solution.

Without getting too technical with the science and terminology, healing DR is a top to bottom issue as discussed. It starts with the way you breathe, the way you stand, and how you move through the exercises. We need to address those issues so your core exercises will be efficient. In addition, healing DR has to do with how your core muscles manage the core pressure.

Everything we do generates core pressure to various degrees, which is there to protect our spines. Some movements create more pressure and some generate less pressure. Progressive Combo Training, with all five fitness elements previously described, will help your core to withstand the various loads that it encounters during a variety of exercises. As you fatigue your core, you will build it up to endure heavier loads in a gradual manner, so the TA muscles and the abdominal wall will be restored.

It is also important to note that it is tough to have a flat tummy by only doing core exercises without doing the other four elements of Progressive Combo Training because you cannot pinpoint or spot treat a specific area for fat loss.

## How Long It Takes to See Changes

Below (figure 7.2) is one of my client's 8-weeks transformation. Trang started with a non-functional 4 fingers and 2 knuckles deep diastasis recti after having 3 babies. After 8 weeks of following these seven secrets above, she was able to bring down the gap to 2.5-3 fingers wide, and 1-1.5 knuckles deep. She also lost 10 lbs during the process.

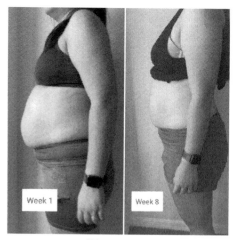

*Figure 7.2*

# Regarding Milk Supply

It is not exercise that causes your supply to decrease, but food and drink consumption. When you work out, you need to eat and drink more. We will talk about DR specific nutrition next.

# Healing Diastasis Recti While Nursing

If you are still in the phase of nursing your baby it will probably take longer to heal your diastasis recti. The hormone relaxin increases the laxity and softness of ligaments. I do not at all suggest that you quit breastfeeding just to heal your DR. If you are a breastfeeding mom, then you know how wonderful breast milk is for your baby. It is much more important to breastfeed your baby than to be in a hurry to heal your DR in my opinion.

# Remember To Always Listen to Your Body

Determining which stage of the DR journey you are in, which targeted exercises are suitable for you, and how well you can handle your intra-abdominal pressure with good posture, will ensure that you can safely do any activity you want.

Finally, before you begin any exercise program, it is vital to perform a pre-activity screening or check with your doctor to ensure that your body is ready to exercise on a regular basis. Do you have any underlying conditions? Do you have a continuous headache, pain, shortness of breath, dizziness or other medical issues? Use your common sense and stop if you feel pain or undue shortness of breath during exercise, or pressure on your pelvic floor.

# Chapter 8:

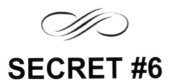

# SECRET #6

## Diastasis Recti-Specific Nutrition

## How Bloating Slows Progress

Think about this: even if you didn't have diastasis recti and you drank beer regularly, you would end up with a beer belly. When you already have diastasis recti, drinking beer would make the belly a lot worse. Your abdominal muscles are already weak, and by adding more pressure from food that produces gas, you will feel ten times more bloated and uncomfortable.

Have you ever seen your belly move by itself like there's an alien inside? It's not an illusion, it's your gas baby. You can literally see the gas travelling down your intestines. It sounds pretty gross, but it's true.

With bloating, whether it is from food or your period, it will be harder for you to contract your abdominal and pelvic floor muscles. Not only that, but you will continue to look pregnant. Hence, even if your only goal is to lose weight, proper nutrition is still as important.

## Food that Make You Gassy

Everyone tolerates food differently. However, here is a list of foods that are common culprits for causing gas and bloating:.

- Foods rich in starch.

- Vegetables such as broccoli, cauliflowers, brussels sprouts, spinach, raw uncooked vegetables which are hard to digest.

- Soda.

- Dairy.

- Beans & lentils.

- Foods high in gluten.

- Red meat.

- Processed foods.

# A Few Tips to Get Started:

1. Keep a food diary. When you are bloated, look back at what you've eaten or drunk in the last few hours – that's when gas typically occurs.

2. Experiment with foods one by one like when your baby starts solids. If you suspect that a particular food will make you bloated, try it, isolate it, and see if it is true.

3. Take your time and gradually add more quantity. If you love red meat and can't live without it, but you know it makes you bloated, then eat a little bit at a time and increase the amount over time.

4. Avoid swallowing air. Eating and talking at the same time, chewing gum, or taking the last sip of a drink using the straw will cause you to suck up a lot of air.

5. Take a supplement that gives you pro- and pre-biotics as well as digestive enzymes.

6. Ensure you are managing and minimizing stress in your life.

7. Eat easy to digest food. Instead of raw salads, try sauté veggies. Instead of nuts, try nut milks. Instead of an unripe fruit, wait until it is ripe to eat.

# A Side Note for Breastfeeding Moms

During the first three months of your baby's life, he or she will go through numerous growth spurts. Your baby may be gassy. When a baby has gas, tiny bubbles develop in their stomach or intestines and it sometimes causes pressure and stomach pain. As a nursing mom, it would be helpful for you to watch what you eat, so you can avoid passing gas-prone foods to your baby through breastmilk.

## Other Ways to Help With Gas

The methods I'm sharing below are old wives' tales passed down from my grandmother's generation! My ethnicity is Chinese, so you may have heard of them, or you may find it super strange! Keep an open mind and see if it works for you!

1. Drink half a tablespoon of fresh minced ginger boiled like a tea first thing in the morning.

2. Soak your feet above your ankles in a hot tub with half a cup of drinking alcohol, or a bunch of maple leaves (yes, you can pick up the leaves in your backyard, but boil them first).

3. Wrap your tummy with a cloth or a belly wrap, so the wind doesn't go into your body through the belly button and rub your belly in a clockwise motion.

## Nutrition and Portion Control

These days everyone is talking about eating clean. We all know that you won't get a flat belly without some food discipline. But what most people aren't talking about is the concept of portion control. Following some latest fad diet won't help you shed the extra pounds, but portion-controlling your food will. You can still enjoy your food without depriving yourself and affecting your breastmilk. Powerful results will happen when you combine it with a superfood protein shake and gas-reducing food.

Let's talk about the important role of nutrition when it comes to healing diastasis recti.

## On the Topic of Counting Calories and Food Tracking

Counting calories is an excellent choice if you are NOT a busy mom! Every time I take my phone out, my toddler snags it from me. Counting calories is so time-consuming and yet such a misleading measure of how healthy your diet is. How much time do you have to calculate the calories in your takeout meal? Is it okay to consume a dozen zero-calorie sodas a day since it adds up to, well, zero calories?

When we resolve to lose weight, what comes to our mind first? Oh we need to cut calories! We need to eat low-fat this and drink low-cal that, or eliminate carbs from our dinner, and count every single bite that goes into our mouth.

You will likely not lose any weight this way, but you'll certainly lose your mind! In addition, if you're breastfeeding, then you won't just deprive yourself but your baby too!

Just carrying a baby around requires a lot of energy, working out means extra nutrition, and most importantly, breastfeeding moms need additional food and water so that their milk supply can meet the needs of their growing baby. We need to learn how to eat healthy, tasty and fulfilling foods so we can stay invigorated and get the results we want.

A healthy and sustainable nutrition approach is not about counting calories or banning foods, it is about how much we eat. It's about eating all the food groups – the right amount of macro and micro nutrients that your body needs so it can absorb and assimilate all the good nutrition.

Everything needs to be fast for moms! I find that portion control is a lifesaver for me. It is so easy to use, so intuitive, so convenient. I am never 'hangry', and I can eat anything.

## Portion Control Containers Systems

I use these six colour-coded rainbow portion control containers to keep track of how much I eat a day. The rule is if it fits, I can eat it.

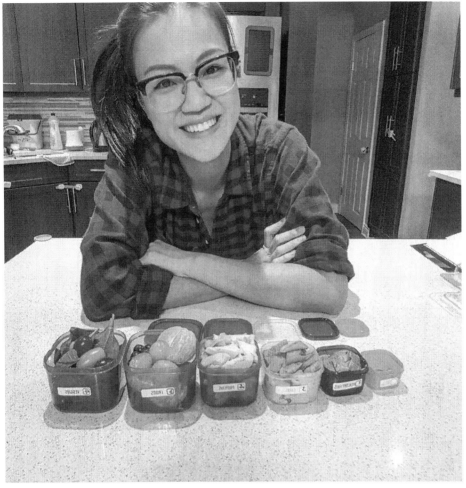

*Figure 8.1: Portion control containers*

In my own example, I do a calorie calculation only once every few weeks. I calculate my calorie target for weight loss (or maintenance), and this is based on my current:

A. weight

B. lifestyle (for example, I'm moderately active).

C. exercise or training program,

D. additional caloric needs (for example if I am breastfeeding, I add 400 calories more to maintain my milk supply).

I calculated that I need 1,778 calories per day. I then translated this calorific need to cover all the food groups using my research, common sense and intuition. It means that every morning I know how many times I can fill each container a day with what type of food

In this example, I need to eat the following numbers of containers in each color:

- 4 x Green - Vegetables

- 3 x Purple - Fruits

- 1 x Blue - Healthy Fats

- 4 x Red - Protein

- 3 x Yellow - Carbs

- 1 x Orange - Seeds and dressing

The containers are 1/2 to 1 cup each depending on which color it is, so it is a lot of food. I am literally eating all day. This system is so simple and easy to use.

You want to find a balanced nutrition regime that fits your lifestyle, so you can stick to it for the foreseeable future. As long as you include all the nutrients and vitamins, and avoid food that makes you gassy, then it is a good diet for YOU. You need energy to work out, you need the vitamins and minerals to help repair the stretched connective tissue in your tummy, you need to fuel yourself and nourish your nursing baby.

Hence, I don't suggest intermittent fasting for breastfeeding women. The keto diet is fine, but it seems very complicated with specific requirements.

Here are some probing questions to help you think about a new diet:

1. Is it easy to meal prep?

2. Are you fueling yourself with all the nutrition and food groups?

3. Can you see yourself sticking to it in the long term?

4. Can you somewhat maintain it even at a restaurant or gatherings?

5. Is it easy to avoid gassy foods?

6. Will you forget to eat?

7. Is it too restrictive?

# Benefits of a Superfood Protein Shake

You need protein to help build muscles, repair tissue, and make enzymes and hormones. You can supplement your dietary protein with protein powder, which may also aid weight loss and help tone your muscles. But when you have a superfood protein shake, you also benefit from all the vitamins, antioxidants, fibre and minerals packed into the powder  thanks to the addition of many different superfoods.

Since your abdominal muscles are made of a structural protein called collagen, eating collagen-rich foods or foods that boost collagen production may help create the building blocks (amino acids) of a strong core. So, what are some of the foods that can help you?

- Fruits such as orange, kiwi, goji berries, and pomegranate are high in vitamin C.

- Kale and matcha are also rich in vitamin C as well vitamin A and antioxidants.

- Nuts, seeds and beans which are sources of zinc.

- Eggs, meats, milk, fish, pea protein (vegan) provide good sources of protein.

- Almonds, grass-fed meat and flaxseed are all rich in Omega 3 which helps the process of regenerating collagen.

- Garlic helps to repair damaged tissue.

- Bone broth is rich in collagen.

It's hard to include so many foods with specific minerals and vitamins in our daily meals. Our grocery bill would be massive, too, if we were to buy them fresh all the time. However, we should endeavour to consume some fresh foods every day, and fill in the gaps with a yummy superfood protein shake to keep us full. Shakes can be a time-saver, and may become a go-to snack--not to mention they can have excellent nutritional value!

As a bonus, some protein shakes have added pre- and pro-biotic digestive enzymes. This may be especially helpful for moms with diastasis recti who often feel bloated, and just need one less thing to think about! The superfood protein shake will help generate new collagen in our bodies, boost our energy and immune system. So, we can be super moms who feel amazing!

We can do the workouts, wear the belly wrap, but **change begins with what goes into your mouth.**

# Chapter 9:

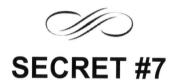

# SECRET #7

## Remain Consistent

If you are still reading this book, I am so proud of you! It shows that you are serious. But most importantly, you want to change more than you want to stay the same. And I know this is YOUR time.

I am not going to sugar coat this one. It is going to take physical and mental work, and being consistent. If you want the results, you have to put in the work.

## Finding Your WHY

Let's figure out what your WHY is? What is the real reason behind your workouts and nutrition? I want you to be very specific with your why.

1. Why do you want to heal your diastasis recti and lose weight?

2. Why is that important to you?

3. How would you feel if you attain it?

4. How would you feel if you don't attain this goal?

5. How would that make your loved ones feel?

6. If you don't do anything or do little about reaching your goal, are you kay with it?

7. If you answer no to question #6, ultimately, why is this goal important to you?

If your reason is 'I want to get rid of the belly so I can fit into my old dress', then your WHY is not strong enough. It is not going to get you through the tough times when you have an unexpected workload, a chaotic weekend, when your kids are not sleeping, or when wine and the couch beckon.

Everyone wants to look good in their clothes, but why is this so important to you? Dig deeper.

For me, I wanted to get rid of the mommy pooch and lose weight, so I could feel confident and fabulous in my clothes. Why? Because I wanted to look presentable when I was with my husband and kids in front of friends and family. Why? So that I could stop being so self-conscious, and focus on the conversation and enjoy the warmth of togetherness. So I wouldn't shy away from social commitments. So I wouldn't start my day feeling gloomy standing in front of my closet. So I could laugh and play and be a whole part of my children's fleeting childhood captured in photos. And most importantly, I wanted to be a role model to my kids, and actively show them that if mommy can achieve her dreams, then they too can achieve anything they want in life.

Do you see how that is a much stronger WHY than just wanting to look good in jeans? Take some time now, and ask yourself those questions above to discover your WHY.

## How Do You Stay Consistent and Motivated

When I first started working out, my daughter was three months old, and my son had just turned two. I was working on my coaching business in small pockets of time through the day, and after they'd gone to sleep at night. You bet being a full-time mom and a CEO mom boss is a 24/7, no sick day, and no vacation day kind of job. I have immense respect for full-time commuting parents of young kids, as it is one of the hardest things one can do. If you're trying to pump at work, doing nursery pickups and drop-offs, in addition to housework, it is very understandable that you feel stretched in a million directions already.

With so much going on, how do you find the time to stay motivated and consistent? I want to share some tips I have learnt through my postpartum journey. Here they are in list form, and expanded on in detail below:

When I first started working out, my daughter was three months old, and my son had just turned two. I was working on my coaching business in small pockets of time through the day, and after they'd gone to sleep at night. You bet being a full-time mom and a CEO mom boss is a 24/7, no sick day, and no vacation day kind of job. I have immense respect for full-time commuting parents of young kids, as it is one of the hardest things one can do. If you're trying to pump at work, doing nursery pickups and drop-offs, in addition to housework, it is very understandable that you feel stretched in a million directions already.

With so much going on, how do you find the time to stay motivated and consistent? I want to share some tips I have learnt through my postpartum journey. Here they are in list form, and expanded in detail below:

1. Choose a program that fits your current life.

2. Make exercise as convenient as possible.

3. Work out when your kids are awake.

4. Exercise around the same time every day.

5. Reward yourself.

6. Expect that your routine will change from time to time.

7. Measure and weigh yourself every week.

## 1. Choose a Program That Fits Your Current Life

As I have mentioned, you need a High-Intensity Total Body Workout. You can sign up for classes at your local gym, get a personal trainer, or you can workout at home with an online coach. There are a variety of programs you can find online.

One thing you want to ask yourself is: what is the length of the program and how long is each session? Is it 4 times a week or 7? (anything less than 4 times a week is probably not going to get you results). Is it 25 or 45 minutes long? Don't forget to count your shower time and commute time if you decide to find a trainer or go to the gym. How long does it take in total?

For example, if you want to go to the gym which is 10 minutes away, class is 40 minutes, you chit-chat with friends for another 10 minutes, shower for another 10 minutes, then come home, then the total estimated time for this exercise is actually 1 hour and 20 minutes.

Can you spare 1 hour and 20 minutes, four times a week outside of your home? If yes, then that's great! If not, then you can work out at home. How do you choose a fantastic at-home program? Refer back to secret #4.

## 2. Make Exercise as Convenient as Possible

Imagine, in the winters it is -20 Celsius or -4 Fahrenheit outside. Would you want to shovel the snow, clear the car and drive to the gym? Make it as convenient as you can. If you go to the gym, go on your way to work, during lunchtime or straight after work.

If you work out at home, designate an area, so you don't have to move furniture around. Keep the laptop or iPad there so you can press play right away. Do an equipment-free or minimal equipment program. In the beginning, you can use water bottles or even your baby as a weight! Make it so convenient that there is no reason for you to not do it.

## 3. Work Out when your Kids are Awake (At home)

A lot of people tell me that they can work out only when the kids are not around. I can tell you right now, that's just an EXCUSE, and I mean it. After working out with an ever-growing baby and a bouncy toddler in my living room, the best motivation is working out when they are awake.

Here are a few reasons why:

1. You will have more energy now than after they go to bed at night.

2. If you try to wait until they nap, they might not nap at all, or if they wake up early you will get frustrated.

3. What's better than involving and letting your children see what mommy is doing? You are not only keeping a promise to yourself, you are also making a promise to your kids by role modelling what consistency and discipline are.

4. It is a time-saver; you kill many birds with one stone. Your kids get to watch an entertaining show of you panting and going up and down! Or they might join you and have great bonding time together, and you get your workout done!

If your baby cries, take it in stride. Carry her in the carrier and work out. If your toddler demands attention, give him something he likes, such as a snack, craft, books etc. They are going to get used to you working out after a few days. Tell them why you are working so hard and what you want to achieve, and I promise they will understand.

If you need inspiration on how it is possible to work out with kids at home, follow my Instagram @beckychoi and watch my stories and highlights. You will know exactly what I mean, so you can do the same!

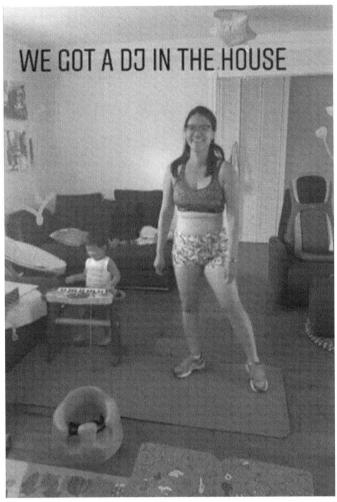

*Figure 9.1: Workout when kids are awake. See Instagram @beckychoi_ for more tips on staying consistent when you have a young family.*

## 4. Make It a Routine to Exercise Around The Same Time

Our brain functions well when there is a routine, so we know what we are expecting next. For example, wake up, breakfast, playtime, lunch, workout, playtime, prep meals, dinner, bath, bed.

It's hard for stay-at-home moms to set rigid minute-by-minute schedules, but I found that if you use breakfast, lunch and dinner as your main time blocks, and tell yourself mentally that you need to work out before lunch, then you will find the time around other errands. This way, it is easy to remember, and it will become a habit, just like a mid-morning coffee.

## 5. Reward Yourself

We all need a little something to motivate us once in a while. Food motivates me a lot, so I always look forward to my peanut butter chocolate protein shake after my workouts! What do you look forward to? If your reward is something that you shouldn't be eating a lot of? Once in a while is still okay but don't go crazy!

## 6. Expect That Your Routine Will Change From Time to Time

You might have to work on projects, so you are coming home late every day. Or your toddler is skipping her nap now, or your schedule changes due to summer break/winter holidays. Anticipate these changes, and see which new time slot you can fit your workout in, and then stick with that time. You might have to do this every few months, and that's okay. This is a healthy lifestyle you are creating, not an overnight success. C'est la vie!

## 7. Measure and Weigh Yourself Every Week

Remember, progress is powerful. A lot of people make the mistake of not measuring or weighing themselves until the end of the program because they don't want to be disappointed. DON'T do that.

Instead of thinking that no change is disappointing, think of it as a moment to reflect. If you didn't lose an inch this week, reflect on what you could have done better. Could you have challenged yourself a little harder? And if you have done your best, that's fine, don't be hard on yourself. Pat yourself on the back knowing that you did everything you could. Hard work never goes to waste. It'll show sooner or later. You should be really proud of yourself. Celebrate the small wins. And trust the process!

## BONUS TIP:

Don't sit down!

How many times have you experienced this? After you come home from a long day at work, or a long day outside with the kids, all you want to do is lie down on the couch and do nothing? This will FOR SURE kill your momentum and motivation. Don't sit; put on some music, drink a high quality, clean energy drink, and go go go!

I have seen many women come into our community, and I've found that there are only two kinds of people. Those who stay committed to their original goals and strive strive strive, and those who are good at making excuses.

The magic won't happen overnight. If you start making excuses (I am tired, I am very busy, I love eating too much), then I hate to tell you thiis, but I think you are going to have a really hard time getting the flat belly and losing weight.

The good news is that you get to choose. In this moment, you can choose which type of person you are going to be. Don't be someone who makes excuses, be someone who actually does what they say they are going to do.

I hope that by knowing your WHY and using the tips mentioned above, you will stay consistent.

## Diastasis Recti Improvement

If you are wondering whether you are making any improvement with the abdominal separation, here are a few ways to track your progress. It can be any of the indications below or a combination of the following metrics:

1. Diastasis recti gap

2. Linea alba depth

3. Your core strength

4. Your midsection measurement when relaxed and when flexed

5. Morning and dinner progression

# 1. Diastasis Recti Gap (width)

The finger gap is a widely used measurement when it comes to progression. If you have a 4+ finger gap, it is ideal to bring it down 1 to 2. However, if you are at a 1 to 2 fingers gap and it is not decreasing, it does not mean that you are not making progress, see metrics #2 to 5.

# 2. Linea Alba Depth

How deep can your fingers sink in? Use the tracker provided in secret #1 for your before and after. Normally, you should expect to see a shallower depth in your diastasis after about one to two months of consistent practice.

# 3. Core Strength

Are you able to maintain tension longer, or with better control while doing the same exercise as last week/month? Are you able to do more advanced moves without compromising alignment and the pressure such as doming, bulging?

## 4. Midsection Measurement

Measure your waist before breakfast, both flexed and relaxed positions, then compare to your previous results.

## 5. Morning and Dinner Progression

Do you feel that your tummy is less bloated after dinner compared to before? Is your stomach less prominent after a meal? A side view picture will help.

Be sure to take notes of these metrics weekly! Tracking keeps you focused on what's important to reach your goals. It also helps you remain motivated and identify potential obstacles. Many people fail to accomplish their goals, not because they don't know how, but they lose sight and go off track.

# Section Three:

# Common Postpartum
# Related Conditions

What if you realize that you have DR, and you don't actively plan on healing it because of lack of time, underlying health issues, monetary constraint, or personal circumstances. What might be the consequences of living with DR, like the previous generations did?

Have you ever noticed how your grandmother has or had this soft, cuddly belly, perhaps bulging forward? Mine did. Back in the day, our grandparents usually had quite a few babies; my grandmother had six! You can imagine how her belly must've expanded and contracted six times (what a miracle!). Thus, her core muscles, combined with the loose skin and excess fat on her abdominal wall, lost normal strength and tone. Back then, no one expected new mothers to 'bounce back' to their pre-baby shape. A bigger, saggier, flabbier postpartum body was accepted just fine, and you went on with life.

So why does it seem like diastasis recti has suddenly surfaced out of nowhere in the last decade? Well, we live and we learn. Your grandmother probably wasn't popping prenatal vitamins, and also didn't know that she might have had diastasis recti. The latest science and research continue to bring more awareness to professionals everywhere. My grandmother was busy taking care of her household and six young children, never mind diastasis recti. By the time her children grew up, she was already in her late 40s. The bulge and her appearance weren't her priority, but how did it affect her functionally, her core and pelvic strength?

Aside from the aesthetic aspect, we need to think of the bigger picture in terms of function. If diastasis recti is left untreated, it can lead to back pain, urinary incontinence, hernia, and inability to perform regular exercises, as we have already discussed. You might be experiencing some, or none of these issues now, but what may happen five, or ten, or even thirty years down the road?

In the next several chapters, we will discuss some postpartum conditions commonly seen in moms with diastasis recti, and finally, we will discuss when you may need surgery and what to consider.

# Chapter 10:

# Uterine Prolapse

When I was pregnant, I remembered my mother would tell me not to take the stairs nor walk around, especially during the first few weeks after childbirth. She even told my husband to carry me up 13 flights of stairs to my bedroom after coming home from the hospital. I had no clue why she suggested it, and I thought it was another old wives' tale. She mentioned that something inside my vagina could fallout if I wasn't careful! Later, I realized she was talking about prolapse.

The uterus is held in place by pelvic muscles and ligaments or the pelvic floor. Uterine prolapse occurs when the muscles become so weak and stretched that they can't support the uterus. Some women experience it during pregnancy and childbirth. During pregnancy, the baby's weight can put pressure on the internal organs and the pelvic floor causing the bladder, uterus or bowel to shift from their normal position.

## Symptoms and Remedies

Some prolapse symptoms include urinary incontinence, a bulge or feeling heavy or dragging down in the vaginal area, fecal leakage from the anus, and discomfort during sex.

Your healthcare provider will perform a vaginal physical exam to evaluate the organ placement and vaginal tone. In more severe cases, an ultrasound or MRI will help determine the stage of the prolapse.

Many women find pelvic floor exercises such as Kegels treat the mild form of uterine prolapse. A study shows that women who regularly do their pelvic floor exercises have a higher chance of healing. They can prevent the deterioration of prolapse and decrease the severity and frequency of symptoms caused by it.

However, in more severe cases, doctors will recommend medical treatment such as a vaginal pessary, which is a vaginal device that supports the uterus and keeps it in position, or a surgical repair.

## Prevent a Prolapse during Pregnancy

There is no guaranteed way to prevent a prolapse while pregnant as it could be caused by a difficult vaginal birth, delivering multiple babies, or other pre-existing health conditions.

If you're planning for a baby or are currently pregnant, seeing a qualified physiotherapist will be able to help you decide what option of preventive measure is suitable for you.

As your body changes and realigns during pregnancy, keeping fit throughout your pregnancy can reduce your risk of prolapse after birth. Therefore, pelvic floor exercises are very beneficial, and I will list some of those exercises in the next chapter.

Take the time you need to do your pelvic floor exercises, walk and stay fit. The stronger your core muscles and pelvic region are, the better off you'll feel during pregnancy. Also, you are likely to be able to rebuild your core faster after childbirth.

# Chapter 11:

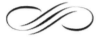

## Pelvic Floor Exercises

Pelvic floor exercises are beneficial, with or without pregnancy. Pelvic floor exercises are exercises that keep your muscles toned within your pelvic region. They are usually done while lying supine on the floor but can be done sitting as well.

## The Importance of Pelvic Floor Exercises

Pelvic floor exercises are important because when you are pregnant, there is added pressure in the abdominal region that can strain your pelvic floor muscles. Without proper care, these muscles can become weak. Weak pelvic floor muscles can cause incontinence and other problems, such as a prolapse discussed in the last chapter.

Pelvic floor muscles play the following roles:

1.  Help you enjoy pain-free sexual intercourse.

2.  Support your spine.

3.  Create a healthy bladder control.

4. Give support to your internal organs (bladder, uterus and intestines).

# Locate Your Pelvic Floor Muscles

Your pelvic floor is located at the base of your pelvis and is the body of muscles attached to your tailbone in the back and your pelvic region in the front. These muscles then connect to the sides of your pelvis where you sit.

Finding your pelvic floor muscles can be done in a variety of ways. You can learn about your own body by placing one or two fingers in your vagina and squeezing to feel it directly. You can also try squeezing your partner during sexual penetration. Other ways include trying to stop urinating mid-flow occasionally, imagining picking up a blueberry with your lady parts, or imagining a zipper zipping upwards slowly from your pubic bone.

# Pelvic Floor Exercises

## Kegel Exercise

To work weak pelvic floor muscles, lie down or sit with knees slightly apart. First, take a deep 360-degree inhale, and then clench your anal region as if you are stopping yourself from breaking wind as you exhale. Second, take another 360-degree inhale and squeeze your vaginal region for one to two seconds while you exhale. Third, take another big inhale, exhale and squeeze both regions together and hold for a few seconds, and release.

Can you feel the contraction in the front versus in the back? Can you feel the contraction and relaxation? Remember, this is the same technique as engaging the lower TA muscle. It is about mind-to-muscle connection.

The more you contract and relax, the more your muscles will adapt, and it will start to listen to your cues on demand. Kegels are discreet exercises, so it allows you to work your muscles even while watching television, waiting in the grocery store line, or stopping at the traffic light. You will want to do this several times a day and about ten reps each time.

Your goal is to lift and contract your pelvic floor muscles, focusing only on tightening that area without flexing the abdominal muscles. If holding for a couple of seconds becomes too easy, try holding up to ten seconds and working your pelvic floor muscles daily.

However, I would caution that doing too much Kegels may not be the right method for you. You want to establish a natural bodily function. Meaning, you want your muscles to be able to contract and relax on their own. You don't want the pelvic floor muscles to easily lose control, such as with a prolapse, nor to hold tension constantly.

Listen for cues in your body, and ask, am I squeezing too much? Am I doing too many reps to the point that I am unable to relax my pelvic floor easily? Am I doing too much that I have a hard time starting the flow of urine?

## Release Your Pelvic Floor Muscles

If you have done too many Kegels previously or have a tight pelvic floor, you may find your pelvic muscles become overactive. A tight pelvic floor is called the hyperactive pelvic floor instead of the hypoactive pelvic floor described above.

Hyperactive pelvic floor symptoms include pelvic pain, difficulty in starting the flow of urine, pain or heaviness during insertion of a tampon or sex, a sense that the bowel was not empty after a bowel movement, or butt gripping all day.

If you experience any of the symptoms, proper care such as pelvic floor release with breathing work and stretches may be necessary. It is also important to note that you are not squeezing your pelvic floor with maximum force when engaging your transverse abdominal muscles. It should only be about 50-70 percent, otherwise, you may overwork your pelvic floor, causing it to be hyperactive, or other muscles such as the oblique or upper abs will take over the core work instead of your TA muscle.

Remember, the pelvic floor muscle workout routine is not about quantity. It is much better to focus on quality and doing a few rather than rushing through the exercises. Take your time, feel your body and make sure you are getting the results you desire.

While pregnant, it is a good idea to do pelvic floor exercises a couple of times a day. And when you have diastasis recti, knowing whether you have a hypoactive or hyperactive pelvic floor is part of knowing your body, so you are not putting undue pressure on it.

If you are unsure whether you have a tight or loose pelvic floor, consult a women's health physiotherapist, as she will be able to assess you internally and give you the right diagnosis.

# Chapter 12:

# Diastasis Recti vs. Hernia

Diastasis recti and a hernia are two distinctly different conditions, but they are often confused. As we have discussed, DR usually occurs naturally, and it is commonly found in women following a pregnancy.

With DR, it is a widening and thinning of the linea alba (figure 12.1), but your linea alba stays intact in one piece. However, a hernia is when you have a hole in the connective tissue where an internal organ has pushed through. It usually does not hurt when it is touched in the early phase. Therefore, most people don't realize that they have a hernia. Later, it will become more visible when you cough and sneeze, and it can become painful.

In either case, if you discover that you may have a hernia, see a doctor as soon as possible. If left untreated, it can lead to hernia strangulation, which is a very serious condition. However, a hernia can also be asymptomatic, in which case one can function normally with it. If it doesn't create any issues or limit the way you move, exercise or go about your daily tasks, self-monitoring and self-awareness are vital to ensuring a hernia doesn't cause problems.

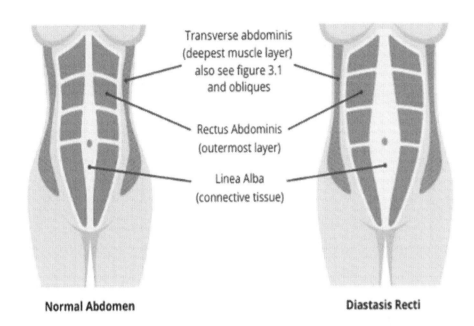

Figure 12.1

# What Are the Symptoms of A Hernia

Some of the symptoms of a hernia are:

1. A bulge or lump when you cough, and it may disappear when you lie down.
2. A popped-out belly button.
3. The bulge has a burning sensation.
4. Pain and discomfort around the bulge area.

5. Weakness in the area.

You need to understand that even though diastasis recti and hernia are two different conditions, they can happen simultaneously. A common postpartum hernia for someone who has DR is umbilical hernia.

An umbilical hernia occurs when some abdominal content, such as your intestine, protrudes through the umbilical hole. When your muscle that holds organs in place becomes too weak, such as in the case of DR, a bulge of organ tissue will push through the abdominal muscle wall.

In my interview with Munira, I asked her if it is possible to get a strong core through exercises when you have a hernia. She said:

> *"100 percent it is. Your core strength can be built within the tissue even if there is a hernia, so it is not going to inhibit someone's progress. One of the jobs of the transverse abdominal muscle, and why it is so important if you have a hernia, is to learn how to strengthen the TA and how to use it, because the TA pulls in against the hernia pressure."*

She also mentions that by learning how to turn on the TA muscles in different positions and movement, you are creating an environment that can be more supportive.

## Umbilical Hernia Treatment

Treating umbilical hernia follows the same principle we talked about in the previous sections – you want to learn how to use our core to contain intra-abdominal pressure. For example, if you anticipate that you are about to squeeze or cough, you want to activate the TA muscles so you can help support the hernia at that moment. If you are exercising, what particular moves are so hard for your core that they create unmanageable intra-abdominal pressure?

A hernia is not something that can be repaired naturally through exercises. It needs to be removed surgically. diastasis recti, which is the thinning and stretching of the linea alba, an umbilical hernia punctures a hole through the abdominal wall (linea alba) near the navel, so exercises will not be able to fill the hole.

If you have a hernia and find that it suddenly becomes more painful than usual, swells up or becomes engorged, you should immediately seek medical attention.

## Cosmetic Aid

You might be wondering what may be useful to help protect the hernia. It's in a secret we have discussed! You got it; it's wearing a belly wrap! Not only will it gently press and counteract the sudden rise in the intra-abdominal pressure such as coughing, but it will also help cover the protruded belly button so that it won't stick out from under your clothes. It will also help support your belly. You can also try wearing high-waisted pants that cover your belly button, similar to maternity pants, but not as high. I would caution you not to wear something too tight with high waist pants that will dig into your belly. Because if it digs into your stomach, it will interfere with your breathing and your hernia.

Remember, when you have both an umbilical hernia and diastasis recti, it is doubly essential to rebuild your core muscles. A strong core will ensure your body can be fully functional for everyday tasks, while also ensuring any hernias you have remain supported.

# Chapter 13:

# Caesarean Scar Issues & Massage

In the last two decades, caesarean surgeries have skyrocketed. Some of these caesarean section surgeries are for health reasons, while others are scheduled for convenience or subsequent caesarean. Either way, caesarean surgery cuts through core muscles and needs to be followed up with care to heal properly.

## Common Caesarean Scar Issues

According to the Canadian Institute for Health Information (CIHI), 28.2 percent of births were via caesarean section in 2018. It is no wonder that issues with caesarean scars have become a topic of concern. The most common way for physicians to perform a caesarean is to do an abdominal incision and a uterine incision, which is usually an incision right above the bikini line in a horizontal manner. The outward scar is just the tip of the iceberg for many women.

After a caesarean, some women have trouble bending, stooping or picking up their newborns because of the pain and discomfort the scar leaves. Others may feel the scar area is too tender to touch. The scar may pull on other muscles nearby and cause lower pelvic pain. Some women find themselves bending forward because of the discomfort, which can cause lower back pain.

Many women are wary of practicing various DR and breathing exercises because they fear that the movement will stretch the scar tissue and cause more tenderness.

Another complication that can be even worse is when the ligament from the labia crosses over the pelvic brim gets caught up in the scar tissue. The tightness can cause significant discomfort and pain when changing positions from sitting to standing.

Women may also experience irritable bowel syndrome, constipation and digestive problems. These types of complications occur when the scar tissue pulls on the abdominal cavity and affects the organs.

## Caesarean Scar Affects the Healing of Diastasis Recti

Your core is made of multiple layers of tissue, so after an incision is made, the process of healing might adhere some layers of tissues together. The adhesion will affect your ability to contract your lower abdominal muscle. And as you recall from secret #1, we need to work on contracting and activating the TA.

Hence, you want the layers of fascia or connecting tissue to glide and move on its own, so you can activate your TA and avoid the complications mentioned above. Strengthening your deep core muscle with breathing exercises will help caesarean recovery as well.

## Caesarean Scar Massage

Recent studies have shown that massage and manipulation of the scar tissue support healthy healing. These days, many physiotherapists help cesarean section mamas heal quicker by getting the incision site to move and increase blood circulation. If you cannot see a physiotherapist, you can try releasing the scar tissue yourself at home.

I understand that because the scar tissue is already painful or tender, many women can shy away from the treatment. However, the gain is worth the pain in most instances, and it isn't always painful.

Don't be afraid to touch and get reacquainted with your body gently. Let it heal for the first four to six weeks postpartum, and try using your fingers to press, softly pinch and roll around the scar. If it is too much for you to handle, wait a day or two, and try again. You don't need to be aggressive with the scar. After all, they are your badges of honour.

# Chapter 14:

# Pregnancy and Diastasis Recti

Too often, pregnancy takes its toll on our routine, and all we want to do is lie in bed and take it easy. The thought of getting up and jumping around, breathing hard, getting all sweaty and tired is just not appealing.

## Pregnancy and Exercise

It is essential to remember that the reward is worth it if you can make it through the first few minutes of fleeting discomfort. Exercise during pregnancy is incredibly helpful and can reduce stress, increase stamina and elevate a mom's mood. Plus, moms who work out tend to have a lower risk of gestational diabetes and preeclampsia. Regardless of the exercise, you should consult with your doctor before beginning a workout routine.

My suggestion is that if you have never worked out before, then don't start something new now. Stick to walking, postural and breathing exercises, and progressively increase the intensity if needed. If you have always been working out, you can most likely maintain what you were doing, but less intensive. And listen to your body. Don't push yourself, do NOT hold your breath, and don't ignore any unusual symptoms.

## Posture during Pregnancy

As your baby grows and your body expands, your posture will change. Proper positioning during daily activities will help ease back pain and other discomforts during pregnancy. Daily stretching will help prevent the high arch on your back, circulate the blood flow and ease your discomfort.

## Prevent Diastasis Recti during Pregnancy

According to research, 100 percent of expecting moms experience diastasis recti if they carry their baby to their due date. There is no prevention; however, they can help prevent the severity of the diastasis. Since the transverse abdominal muscles are responsible for holding our posture and wrap everything in place, working on activating the TA prevents it from becoming slack and underused. Another area to work on is postural exercises, where the focus is breathing into your back so that your back is not excessively curved.

The exercises will help you transition to a full routine after the baby arrives so that you can heal your diastasis recti faster.

# How Kegel Exercises Help During Pregnancy

Kegel exercises help strengthen the vaginal muscles and the pelvic floor muscles that support the uterus, bladder, urethra and rectum. Exercising these muscles not only keeps them toned, but it also improves circulation through the organs that are so vital to a healthy and comfortable pregnancy.

One of the main ways Kegels help during pregnancy is that you become more aware of the location and function of the pelvic floor muscles and how to control them. This may result in more natural labour and delivery.

Please refer to pelvic floor exercises in the previous chapters for more information.

# Chapter 15:

# Diastasis Recti Surgery

After my first DR diagnosis, I remember asking my doctor what the diastasis recti operation, commonly known as the tummy tuck, is actually like. She said, 'You will have to go under general anesthesia. It's a direct invasive repair in which they go through multiple incisions to sew the muscle back together with a mesh. And it will take at least six weeks to recover afterwards.' At that point, thinking about the muscles being stitched back together, I almost threw up.

I said, 'NO WAY that I am doing surgery! What is so hard about healing DR anyway? I am going to fix this stomach myself!' And that was the pivotal point in my life and career.

## The Reasons to Consider a Tummy Tuck Surgery

I learnt about surgery a few years ago; the technology may have improved now with a less invasive repair that achieves the same result. Consult with your surgeon if you are considering surgery.

Here are a few reasons why one would choose surgery and my candid thoughts on each:

1. You feel deeply unhappy about your physical appearance. It's taking a toll on your mental health and intimate relationship.

Imagine you can barely look in the mirror, you stand by the closet for an hour looking for something to wear, and you can't even hug your partner comfortably. And the awful feeling you get when people ask you when you are due. I get it. It's difficult and affects our health as we have to battle and put up with this turmoil every day.

2. You have seen multiple physiotherapists for your diastasis, you have worked with a DR fitness specialist, and you see little to no improvement.

According to my mentor, Dr. Sarah Duvall, it can take a whole year, and even up to two years, to heal your diastasis recti with the right exercise. It can be a long recovery time for some moms. If your work or the sport you play requires you to use a significant amount of core strength and don't want to wait for a year, surgery will speed up the process for you.

3. You have an underlying issue, that if you don't surgically repair your DR, another serious health issue may arise.

I know a mama who is currently battling this. It is not an easy decision. Because of her severe diastasis recti, she has been cornered into deciding that she either get the surgery right away or risk her spine in the future.

# Surgery Considerations

If you opt for surgery, here are some considerations to help you with the budget, give you the real picture, and set you up for success and recovery.

## 1. It's expensive! Anywhere from $5,000 to $15,000

Since it is a major surgery with general anesthesia, you can expect that depending on the severity of your DR. If you also need to repair your hernia, it can get quite expensive. It also depends on the surgeon's experience. In my province in Canada, severe cases are covered by our public health insurance, but others are not covered and are considered cosmetic surgery. Research to see if your case is covered by your insurance or not.

## 2. Is weight loss also your goal?

Most moms usually have some weight they want to lose. But if you are back to your ideal weight and you don't want to lose weight in the near future, then you have an advantage in getting the surgery now. Because surgery can help you pull the muscles back together and lessen the loose skin, but it won't help with your belly fat.

## 3. Your post-surgical abdomen will not look like your pre-baby abdomen.

If you want to get a tummy tuck because you want to look great in your bikini or sports bra or tank, then you might be disappointed. It depends on how they are going to stitch, where the incisions are, and whether you have an umbilical hernia, the scar could be higher or lower. Discuss your particular case with your surgeon in great detail to avoid any surprises.

## 4. You should be done with having babies.

I ruled out surgery immediately when I first heard of it (although I never intended to get one) because I need to be done with having babies. I knew I wanted to have two, maybe three babies in the future, so having the surgery would've halted entirely any hope of that. Because when your belly expands again, guess what will happen to the mesh they put inside?

## 5. The road to recovery is long, and it's even longer in the unfortunate event of an infection.

You are looking at anywhere between 2-3 months minimum for a full recovery. The first few weeks will be the toughest; with tubes attached to your abdomen, you'll be on bed rest, you won't be able to do your daily tasks or lift your kids. So be sure to have enough support around the house and a solid arrangement for child care. You will also want to take proper care of the incision area as you don't want to risk an infection. Above all, give yourself grace. Nothing is more important than taking care of your health after surgery so you come back more robust and happier.

## 6. You still need to learn how to strengthen your core and exercise correctly.

Some moms think that once they do the surgery, they can use their core as usual again. But that's far from true. You need to build your core strength again. You will still need to learn how to 360-degree breathe, engage your TA, align your body and exercise correctly, like you would if you wanted to heal your DR without surgery. Reviewing secrets #1 to #7 and implementing them will help you get the dream body you want faster.

# Section Four: Conclusion

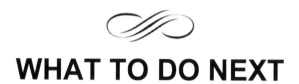

# WHAT TO DO NEXT

## You made it!

I am sure that right now, you probably feel like you have just been through labour once again, and I totally understand that. I really wished that someone told me about diastasis and how to heal it the correct way during my first pregnancy. It probably would have been a much easier road to combat this mummy tummy. However, I believe that everything happens for a reason. I have been blessed with a gift to share with moms like you.

The concepts I've laid out here are thoroughly researched, and tried-and-tested tips and tactics that I use for all my clients. It's taken me years of research and thousands of dollars spent in different programs and consulting other health professionals. Most importantly, I went through this twice after two pregnancies with a lot of trial and error. I hope that instead of feeling overwhelmed, you will realize that the techniques and secrets I have shared in this book are actually a clear and direct route to healing DR.

I understand that everyone's situation is unique. I have shared in these pages only that which has proven to work repeatedly. You can have faith that this will work for you, too.

If you are wondering where you should start, check out the next pages for a 'Quick Start Guide' with a summary of steps.

I hope that reading this book has been an excellent investment of your time. I wrote it with the sincere desire to convey a clear and concise message for you. But no matter how much you read it, you need to take action today.

I once attended a summit, where bestselling author Rachel Hollis said,

*"Knowledge Is Power."*

*WRONG!*

*Applied Knowledge Is Power.*

You need to take what you have learnt and apply it, or else it is garbage.

If you'd like to work closely with me and have me as your coach, this is your invitation! I'm deeply passionate about helping moms with diastasis recti. Severe DR usually requires more attention and care because of how stretched out the entire abdominal wall is. Working with me will speed up the time you spend trying to understand and troubleshoot things. Your program will be customized, streamlined and keep evolving as you go from strength to strength. I will personally hold you accountable. As you see yourself progress and transform, you will be more motivated and consistent, so you can get a strong core faster and rock your little dress! Email me for more information at becky@beckychoi.com or follow me on Instagram @beckychoi

I can't wait to learn more about you and your kids, and be your cheerleader, a friend and a coach.

Thank you so much for spending this time with me. It's truly been an honour. I look forward to witnessing your transformation. I know, you are going to be an aspiring role model for your children, and you ARE a true Tummy Warrior! Come and say hi to me on my social media platform, and please share with me how these secrets have transformed your life.

I'll talk to you soon!

Becky Choi

'It's time to change, mama!'

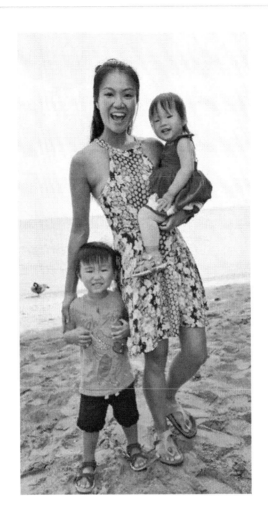

# Did You Enjoy Reading This Ebook?

If so, leave a comment and review on Amazon kindle now. Your review will help shine a light for many other moms experiencing diastasis recti who are desperately searching for a complete solution.

# A Quick Start Guide:

Congratulations on finishing this book! It's important to know that every exercise can become your core exercise. It's not a matter of which 'DR labelled' exercise you do, it's how you do it and how your body reacts. This education will come in handy for a long, long time!

Here's your quick start guide –

1. Determine whether you have any underlying conditions such as a hernia, pelvic prolapses or other medical conditions with a women's health physiotherapist.

2. Check with your doctor to see if you are okay to start a new fitness routine.

3. Take your waist, gap and depth measurement.

4. Learn how to 360-degree deep breathe.

5. Learn how to engage your transverse abdominal muscles.

6. Determine what stage you are at (beginner, intermediate or advanced), and start doing stage-appropriate core exercises and progressively challenge yourself.

7. Pick a total body workout program, pick your meal plan and go through with the program from start to finish.

8. Have fun and enjoy the process. Your consistency can change your life forever.

# References

1. JB Sperstad, MK Tennfjord, G Hilde et al, 'Diastasis recti abdominis during pregnancy and 12 months after childbirth: prevalence, risk factors and report of lumbopelvic pain', *British Journal of Sports Medicine*, 2016.

2. Patricia Goncalves Fernandes, Augusto Gil Brites Andrade et al, 'Prevalence and risk factors of diastasis recti abdominis from late pregnancy to 6 months postpartum, and relationship with lumbo-pelvic pain', *Manual Therapy*, February 2015.

3. Charlotte Hilton Andersen, 'What Is a Postpartum Corset and Should You Try It?', *What to Expect*, 10 July 2018, https://www.whattoexpect.com/wom/baby/the-pros-and-cons-of-wearing-a-postpartum-corset.aspx

4. Munira Hudani, Registered Physiotherapist, Pelvic Health/Women's Health Physiotherapist, Diastasis Rectus Abdominis Course Instructor. https://www.munirahudanipt.com/

5. Dr. Sarah Ellis Duvall, PT, DPT, CPT, CNC, Core Exercise Solution. https://www.coreexercisesolutions.com/

6. https://www.researchgate.net/publication/314102718_Rando mized_controlled_trial_of_abdominal_binders_for_postoper ative_pain_distress_and_blood_loss_after_cesarean_delivery

7. Kim Smith, 'Why is the C-section rate still climbing in Canada? ', *Global News*, 28 May, 2019 https://globalnews.ca/news/5325680/family-matters-c-section-rate-climbing- canada-birth-health/

8. Rachel Hollis, 'Girls, Wash Your Face', Thomas Nelson, 06 Feb, 2018

9. ACSM's Resources for the Personal Trainer Fifth Edition, Wolters Kluwer, 2018

10. https://www.ncbi.nlm.nih.gov/pmc/articles/PMC5558398/ A comparison between stabilization exercises and pelvic floor muscle training in women with pelvic organ prolapse

# About the Author

Becky was born and raised in Hong Kong. She moved to Vancouver, Canada, as an international student when she was thirteen. Living with various homestay families and earning her first babysitting pay at the age of fifteen, helped her become compassionate, independent and resilient. She has a degree in Economics and Employment Relations from the University of Toronto. Her goal was to become a Human Resources Professional, but she ended up spending ten years in retail banking.

Through her personal experience, she found her true passion in postnatal health and fitness, and she feels utterly grateful to be able to follow her calling. Becky is a Certified Postpartum Corrective Exercise Specialist, Certified Personal Trainer and the founder of Tummy Warrior Method.

Becky enjoys travelling and married her husband, Daniel, in Montego Bay, Jamaica. She loves seafood and Asian cuisine, but fried chicken wings are her favourite. Becky and Daniel live in Toronto with their son Jordan, daughter Emily, and their dogs Pocky and Anna.

Thank you for reading the Diastasis Recti Secrets for New Moms e-book.

Sign up for our exclusive video exercise series and references mentioned in the book to heal your diastasis quicker.

Visit us online at guide.beckychoi.com

Printed in Great Britain
by Amazon

80455898R00100